200 juice diet recipes

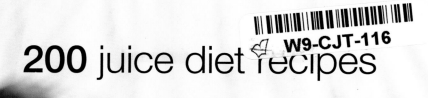

W9-CJT-116

MAY 0 9 2016

641.875 Ski

Skipper, J.
200 juice diet recipes.

PRICE: $9.99 (3559/he   )

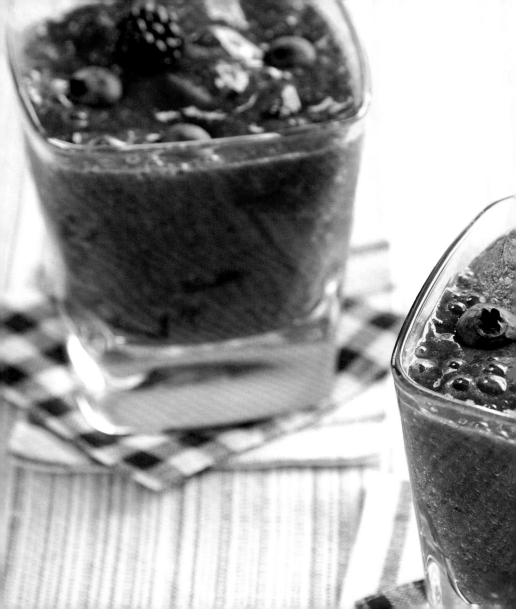

hamlyn | all color cookbook

200 juice diet recipes

Joy Skipper

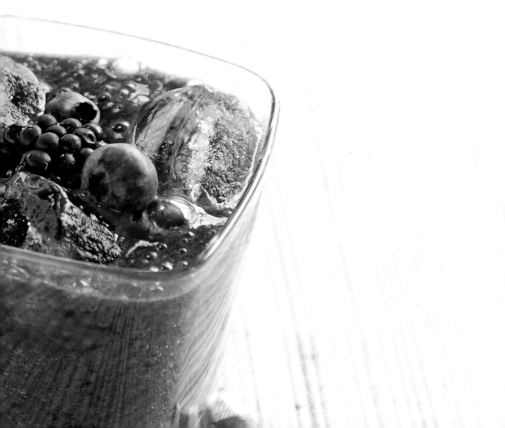

An Hachette UK Company

www.hachette.co.uk

First published in Great Britain in 2015 by Hamlyn, a division
of Octopus Publishing Group Ltd, Carmelite House,
50 Victoria Embankment, London EC4Y 0DZ
www.octopusbooks.co.uk

Copyright © Octopus Publishing Group Ltd 2015

Some of the recipes in this book have previously appeared
in other titles published by Hamlyn.

Distributed in the US by Hachette Book Group,
1290 Avenue of the Americas, 4th and 5th Floors,
New York, NY 10020

Distributed in Canada by Canadian Manda Group,
664 Annette St., Toronto, Ontario, Canada M6S 2C8

All rights reserved. No part of this book may be reproduced
or utilized in any form or by any means, electronic or
mechanical, including photocopying, recording, or by any
information storage or retrieval system, without the prior
written permission of the publisher.

Joy Skipper asserts the moral right to be identified as the
author of this work.

ISBN: 978-0-60063-189-7

Printed and bound in China

10 9 8 7 6 5 4 3 2 1

Standard level kitchen cup and spoon measurements are
used in all recipes unless otherwise indicated.

Scant 1 cup (7 fl oz) makes one average serving.

Ovens should be preheated to the specified temperature;
if using a convection oven, follow the manufacturer's
instructions for adjusting the time and temperature.

Fruit and vegetables are medium unless otherwise stated.

Fresh herbs and freshly ground black pepper should be
used unless otherwise stated.

This book includes dishes made with nuts and nut
derivatives. It is advisable for people with allergic reactions
to nuts and nut derivatives or those who may be vulnerable
to these allergies, such as pregnant and nursing mothers,
people with weakened immune systems, the elderly, babies,
and children, to avoid dishes made with these. It is prudent
to check the labels of all prepared ingredients for the
possible inclusion of nut derivatives.

Before making any changes to your diet and health routine,
always consult a physician.

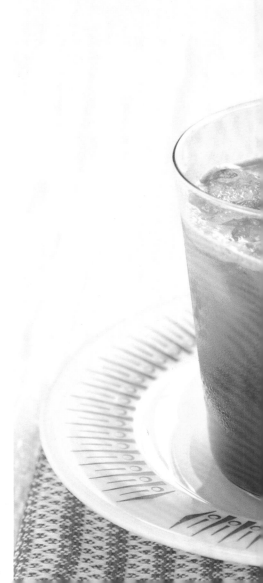

contents

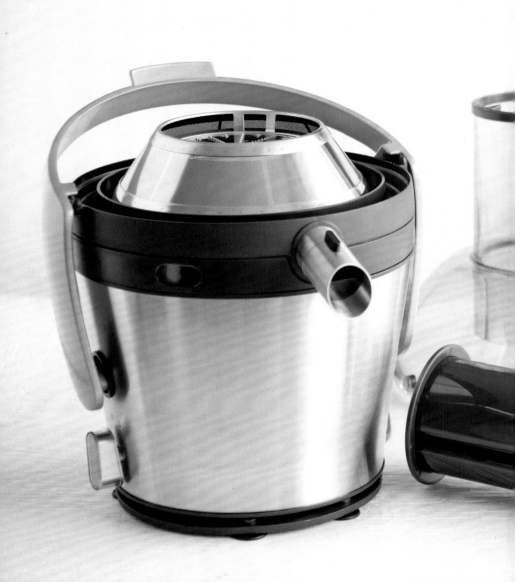

introduction

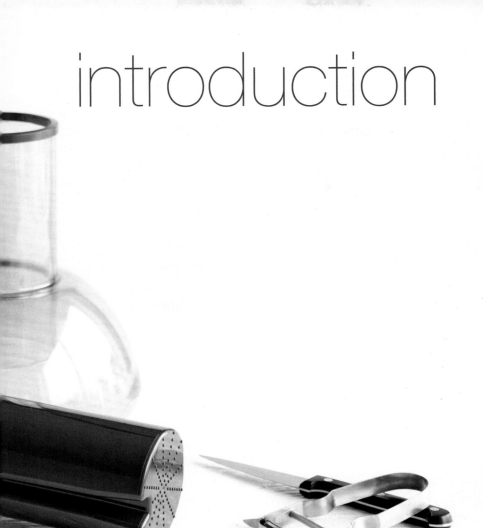

introduction

juicing for diet

One of the easiest ways to improve the nutritional content of your meals is to include juices in your daily diet.

A lot of important vitamins and minerals are found in the fibrous parts of fruit and vegetables, and getting a big hit of those vitamins and minerals would mean eating an enormous amount of food. Could you

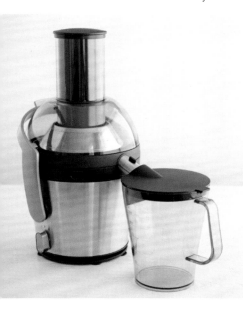

eat two beets, one orange, one apple, half a cucumber, and a wedge of cabbage all in one sitting? Probably not, but you could drink their juice. Juicing releases all the nutrients from those ingredients so that they can be easily absorbed into the bloodstream. We are constantly told to eat more fruit and vegetables, but while eating a large plate of kale for its nutritional content is a tough job, drinking it in a juice with other great-tasting vegetables and fruits is really easy.

Making juices from scratch ensures they are fresh, so it's important to drink them relatively quickly. Once foods have been juiced, the enzymes in the food continue to break down the molecules of food into smaller particles, making the juices easy to digest but with fewer nutrients as time goes by. These enzymes are responsible for hundreds of chemical reactions taking place in our bodies, so including them in our diet is important.

By drinking fresh juices, you help the digestive process, which for a lot of people can be sluggish, and this, in turn, means you will more probably absorb all the great nutrients you consume, which go on to support the other systems throughout your body.

which juicer?

There are two different types of juicer available:

- **Centrifugal**—these are the most common

type of juicer, using a fast-spinning metal blade that spins against a mesh filter, separating juice from flesh via centrifugal force.

• **Masticating**—these juicers extract juice by first crushing and then pressing fruit and vegetables for the highest possible yield.

There are a lot of different models to choose from, so before you rush out to buy one, you need to consider the following questions:

- How easy is it to clean the juicer?
- How small do you have to chop your ingredients?
- How effective is the juicer?
- How much do you want to spend?
- What do you want to juice? If, for instance, you want to juice wheatgrass, you can use only a masticating juicer to do this.

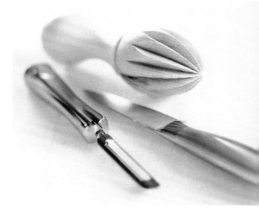

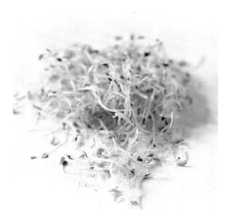

juicing tips

- As with all food preparation, it's good to be organized, so make sure you have all the ingredients on hand before you start.
- The size of the funnel of your juicer will dictate how small you need to chop your ingredients. This is something to take into account when you are choosing your juicer. If the funnel is large enough, you may not need to chop some fruit or vegetables at all.
- You should fill the funnel before starting the juicer and keep the machine running for 15–20 seconds after you have finished juicing. You will be surprised how much juice continues to run out.
- You have to peel ingredients that have thick skin, such as kiwifruit, pineapples,

9

and fresh ginger root. Citrus fruits can be peeled or not; it is entirely up to you.

- If you are juicing a lot of greens, such as spinach or watercress, it's good to add these to the juicer between more solid ingredients, such as apples or carrots, to help them to be pressed into the juicer.
- Because you will be using the peel of a lot of ingredients, be sure to wash the fruit and vegetables thoroughly; even if they are organic, they could still be contaminated with bacteria.
- Wash the juicer immediately after juicing. If you wait too long, the pulp will harden and be difficult to remove.

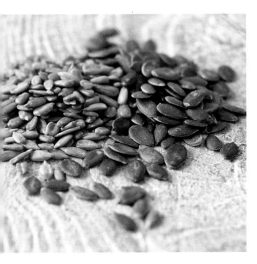

juicing for health

Fruit juices have received a lot of bad press over the past few years, claiming that they are full of sugar and should be consumed in moderation. Well, this is the case for most foods; everything should be consumed in moderation, so keep this in mind when juicing every day.

If you have a sweet tooth or are borderline diabetic, sticking to vegetable juices would be more beneficial for you. If you don't like vegetables, then this is a great way for you to include them in your diet. You will be surprised how sweet the vegetable juices can be (see pages 16–69).

Be aware that drinking too many fruit juices can increase your calorie intake; one small juice could contain three or four whole fruits, so choosing vegetable juices is preferable.

When you juice fruit and vegetables, you remove the fiber, which is necessary for a healthy diet, so it's important to replace the fiber with other ingredients, such as ground chia seeds or ground flaxseed. Alternatively, you could use the pulp from the juicer to make soups or muffins, for example.

juicing for weight loss

When most people try to lose weight, they cut down on a lot of foods, some of which could actually aid weight loss. Reducing

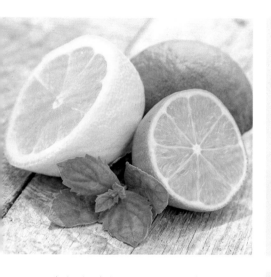

Foods that support the liver

- Garlic
- Grapefruit
- Beet
- Leafy green vegetables
- Avocado
- Cold-pressed oils, such as avocado, flaxseed, and hemp
- Cruciferous vegetables, such as cabbage and broccoli
- Lemons and limes
- Walnuts
- Turmeric

calories tends to mean you are reducing the nutrients that your body needs to run your busy lifestyle. That's where juicing comes in.

There are a number of nutrients that are important when trying to lose weight, mostly those nutrients that support your digestive system (helping you to digest foods and absorb nutrients) and your liver (supporting the detoxification process and getting rid of waste). When you lose weight, you start to lose the toxins that are stored in the fat cells, which gives your liver extra work to do, so supporting the liver at this time is beneficial to your health.

Foods that aid digestion

- Yogurt
- Fish oils
- Ginger
- Pineapple
- Peppermint

is it necessary to fast on juices alone?
Fasting is one way that a lot of people like to start dieting, just because it gives them a boost of confidence when the first weight drops off, but long-term weight loss should be slow and more controlled. Using juices, smoothies, dips, or soups as meal replacements is a better option; the slower you lose weight, the more probable it will be that you keep it off and not experience headaches and withdrawal symptoms while you are doing it. It's also easier to stick to replacing the odd meal than it is to try to fast when you have a busy lifestyle.

Juicing fruit and vegetables is only part of the picture with regards to weight loss; your diet still needs to include both protein and fat.

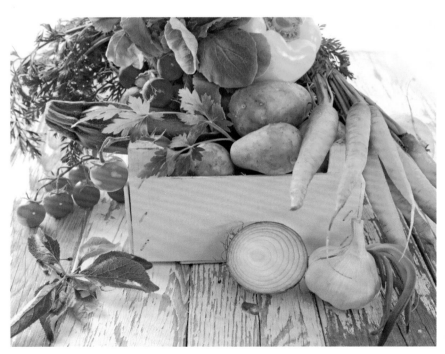

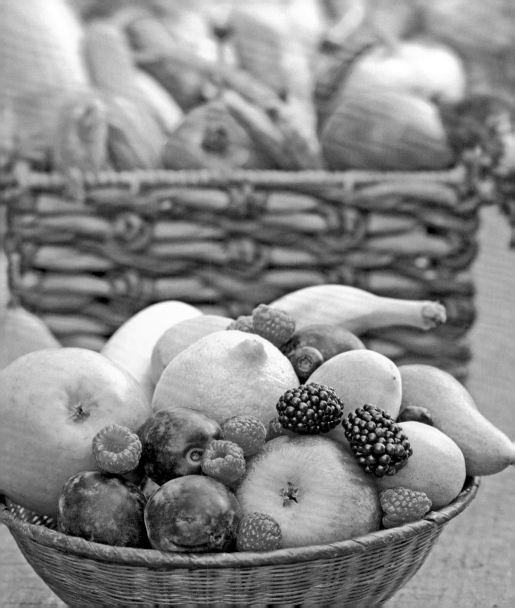

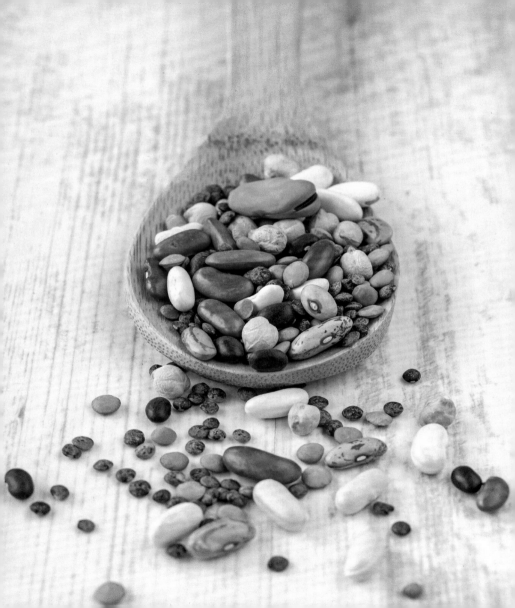

Protein is needed for muscle repair and can be found in lean meats, fish, eggs, lentils and beans, and dairy products. Fat is needed for healthy cells all over the body, including the brain, and good fats are known to help remove bad fats, so you should still include oily fish (such as salmon and mackerel), avocados, and nuts in your diet.

juice diet tips

- Use raw, organic vegetables and fruit wherever possible—to avoid toxins going into your body, you need to eat "clean" foods.

- Limit the number of fruit juices you have each day; choose vegetable juices instead.

- Add protein and fat to your diet by adding chia seeds, flaxseed, avocado oil, protein powder, and green powders, such as wheatgrass, spirulina, and chlorella, to your juices or smoothies.

- Don't drink the same juice every day. As with a normal diet, the more variety, the more nutrients you will probably absorb. Although you have a huge number of recipes to choose from in this book, also experiment with your own combinations of fruit and vegetables.

what about exercise?

Studies have shown that people who lose weight gradually will be able to maintain their weight better with regular exercise. This doesn't mean you need to join a gym. If you've never exercised before, one of the best forms of exercise is walking. Just start to walk for 20 minutes, three times a week, then gradually increase this as you feel you can. When you get to the point that you want more exercise, talk to a personal trainer or ask your local gym for more advice.

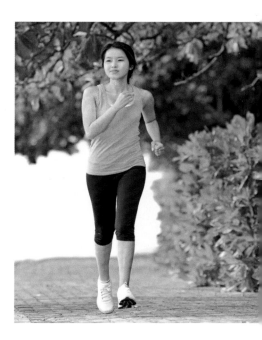

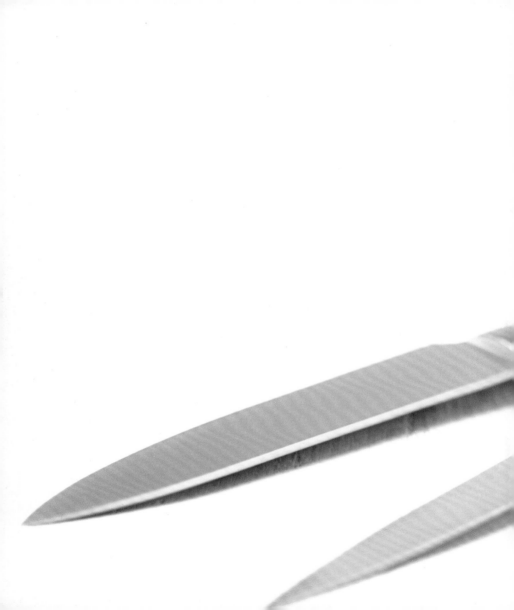

vegetable juices

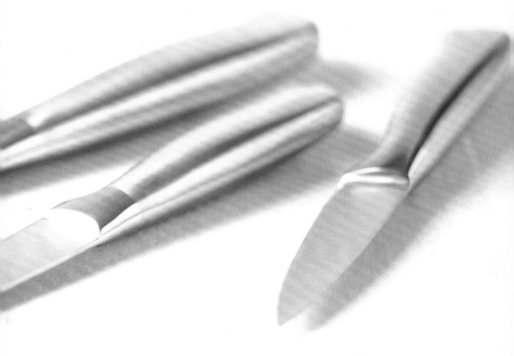

citrus beet juice

Makes **about 1¾ cups
(13½ fl oz)**

1 **orange**
2 small **beets**
2 large **carrots**, plus extra
   to decorate
½ **cucumber**

Coarsely peel the orange. Juice the orange with the beets, carrots, and cucumber.

Pour the juice into a glass, decorate with slices of carrot, and serve immediately.

For spicy citrus beet juice, follow the recipe above, adding a ¾ inch piece peeled fresh ginger root to the juicer with the other ingredients.

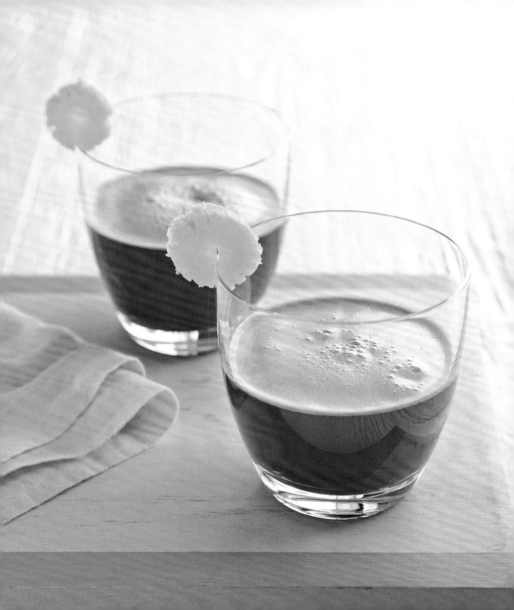

mean green juice

Makes **about scant 2 cups (15 fl oz)**

1 small **apple**
⅓ **cucumber**
2 **celery sticks**, plus extra to decorate
½ cup coarsely chopped **kale**
1 **lemon**
¼ cup **parsley**
1 teaspoon **wheatgrass powder**
ice cubes

Juice the apple with the cucumber, celery, kale, lemon, and parsley. Whisk in the wheatgrass powder.

Pour the juice into a glass over ice, add a trimmed celery stick, and serve immediately.

For sweet mean green juice, replace the kale with an extra apple and 1 orange and juice as above.

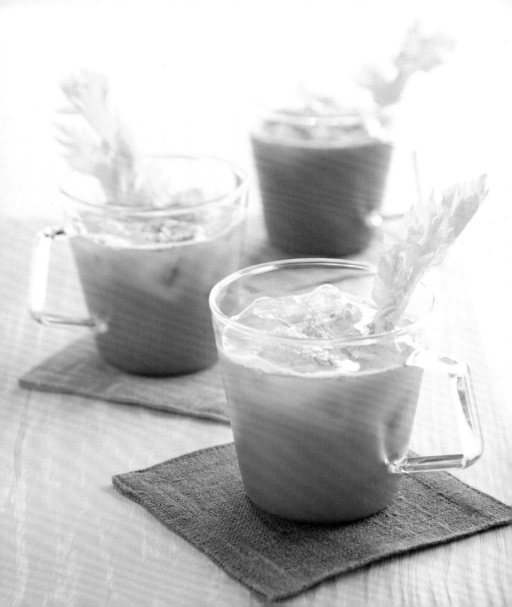

heart beet juice

Makes **about 1½ cups (12 fl oz)**

1 **orange**
2 **beets**
1 small **apple**
ice cubes

Grate the zest of the orange onto a plate. Coarsely peel the orange and cut into wedges. Rub the rim of a glass with a wedge of orange, then dip the rim of the glass into the grated orange zest to coat the rim.

Juice together the orange wedges, beets, and apple.

Pour the juice into the prepared glass over ice and serve immediately.

For green heart beet juice, follow the recipe above, adding 2 cups spinach to the juicer with the other ingredients.

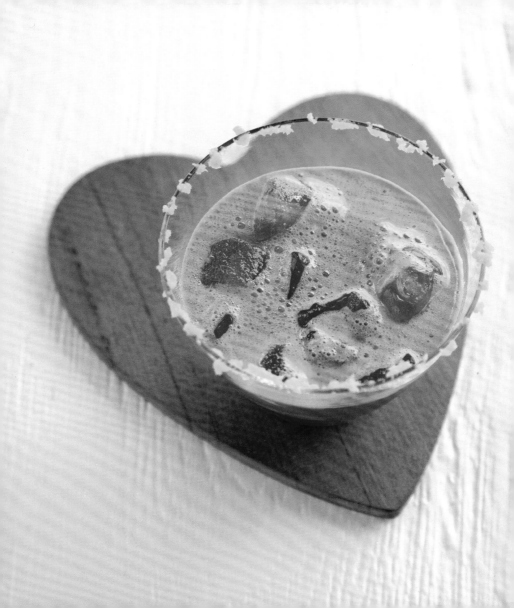

fabulous fennel juice

Makes **about 1¼ cups
(10 fl oz)**

⅔ **fennel bulb**
½ large **apple**
2 large **carrots**
grated **nutmeg**, to sprinkle

Juice all the ingredients together.

Pour the juice into a glass, sprinkle with a large pinch of nutmeg, and serve immediately.

For fennel & orange juice, coarsely peel 1 orange. Juice the orange with ⅔ fennel bulb and 2 large carrots. To add extra fiber to the juice, if desired, stir in ½ teaspoon ground flaxseed.

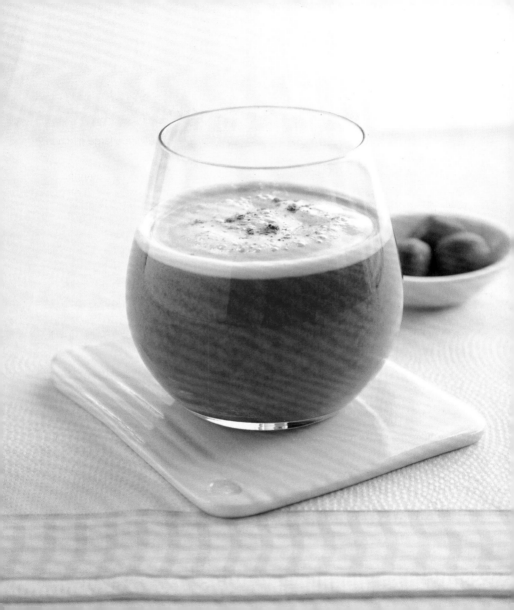

tropical green juice

Makes **about 1½ cups
(12 fl oz)**

⅕ **pineapple**
¾ cup coarsely chopped **kale**
¾ cup **spinach**
1 small **apple**
1 teaspoon **green powder**
  (such as wheatgrass,
  spirulina, or chlorella)
ice cubes

Coarsely peel the pineapple. Juice the pineapple with the kale, spinach, and apple. Stir in the green powder and mix well.

Pour the juice into a glass over ice and serve immediately.

For sweet & hot tropical green juice, replace the spinach with 2 large carrots and juice as above. Stir in a few drops of Tabasco sauce with the green powder and serve poured over ice.

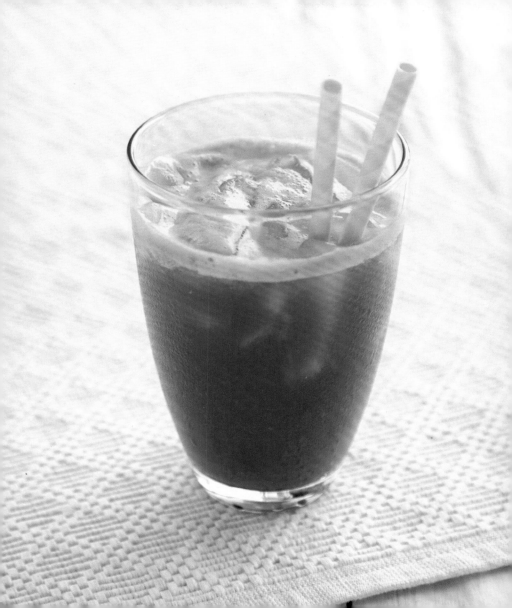

sweet red pepper juice

Makes **about 1 cup (8 fl oz)**

1 teaspoon ground **mixed peppercorns**
lime wedge
1 large **red bell pepper**
20 **red grapes**
2–3 **ice cubes**

Place the ground peppercorns on a small plate. Rub the rim of a glass with the lime wedge and dip the rim of the glass into the peppercorns to coat the rim.

Core and seed the red bell pepper. Juice the bell pepper with the grapes.

Transfer the juice to a food processor or blender, add the ice cubes, and process briefly until smooth.

Pour the juice into the prepared glass and serve immediately.

For hot red pepper juice, core and seed 1 large red bell pepper. Juice the bell pepper with ⅔ small apple and a ¾ inch piece peeled fresh ginger root. Serve with a dash of Tabasco sauce.

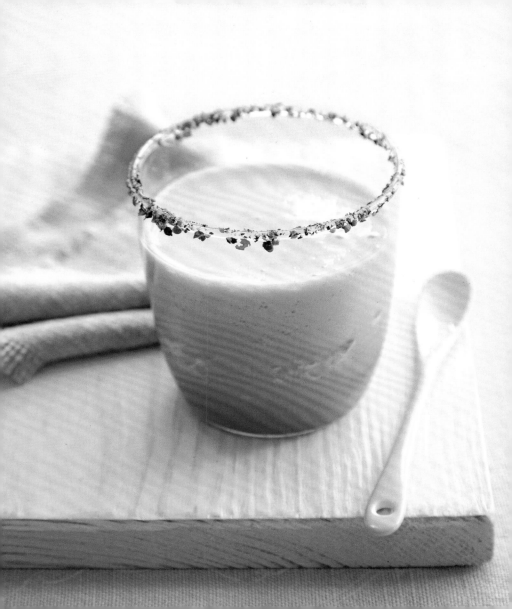

jump-start juice

Makes **about 1½ cups
(12 fl oz)**

1 **lemon**
¾ inch piece fresh **ginger root**
1 **garlic clove**
⅔ small **apple**
2 large **carrots**
2 **celery sticks**
3 cups **alfalfa sprouts**

Coarsely peel the lemon, ginger, and garlic. Juice all the ingredients together.

Pour the juice into a glass and serve immediately.

For clean start juice, juice 1 coarsely peeled lemon with 1 coarsely peeled lime, ½ cucumber, and a ¾ inch piece peeled fresh ginger root. Pour the juice into a tall glass and fill with sparkling water.

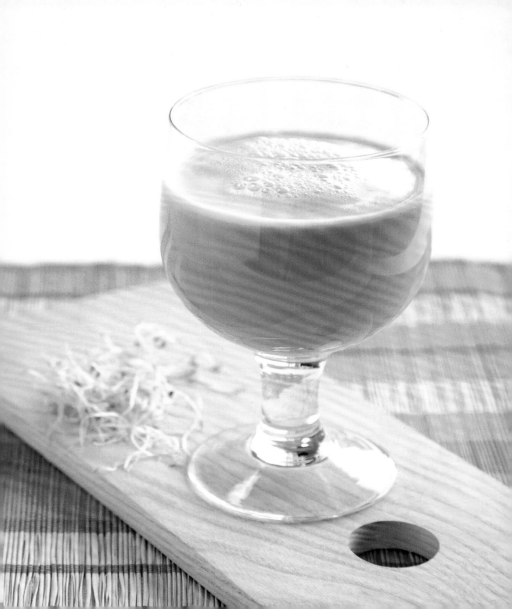

popeye power juice

Makes **about 1 cup
(8 fl oz)**

2¼ cups **spinach**
2 **celery sticks**
⅔ small **apple**

Juice all the ingredients together.

Pour the juice into a glass and serve immediately.

For extra Popeye power juice, juice the spinach, celery, and apple as above, then stir in ½ teaspoon green powder and 1 teaspoon avocado oil and serve.

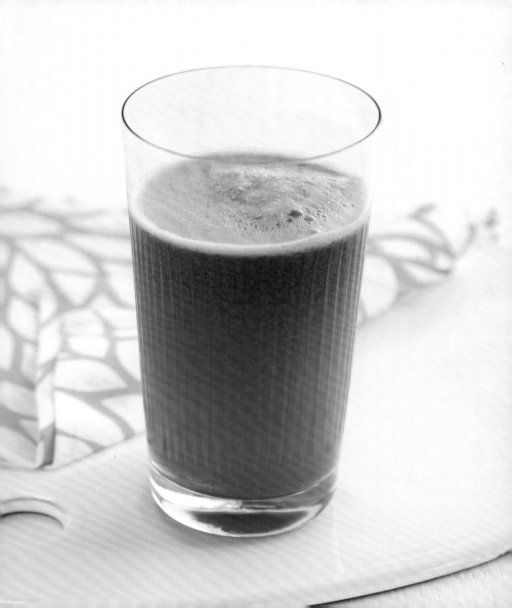

spicy beet juice

Makes **about 1 cup**
(8 fl oz)

2 **beets**
⅓ cup **cilantro leaves**
2 **celery sticks**
large pinch of ground **turmeric**
black pepper

Juice the beets with the cilantro and celery. Whisk in the ground turmeric. Season the juice to taste with black pepper.

Pour the juice into a glass and serve immediately.

For spicy roots juice, juice 1 parsnip, 2 large carrots, ⅔ small apple, and a ¾ inch piece peeled fresh ginger root. Whisk in large pinch of ground turmeric and serve.

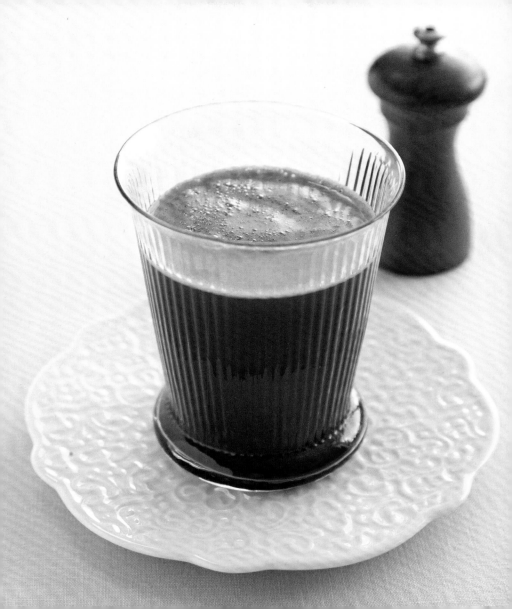

carrot juice

Makes **about 1¼ cups**
(10 fl oz)

1 **lemon**
2 large **carrots**,
2 **Boston** or other small
butterhead lettuce
⅔ small **apple**
1 teaspoon **chia oil**

Grate the lemon zest and reserve. Coarsely peel the lemon. Juice the lemon with the carrot, lettuce, and apple. Stir in the reserved grated lemon zest and chia oil.

Pour the juice into a glass and serve immediately.

For stinging carrot juice, coarsely peel 1 lemon. Juice the lemon with 4 large carrots, ⅔ small apple, and a handful of stinging nettles.

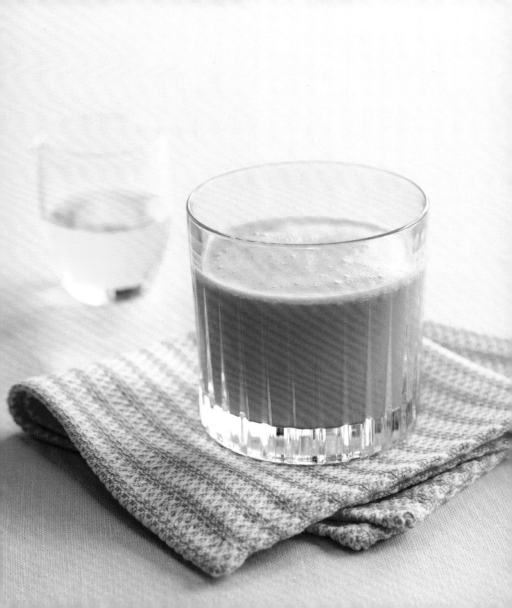

healing green juice

Makes **about scant 2 cups (15 fl oz)**

generous ½ cup coarsely chopped **kale**
1¼ cups **spinach**
1 **Boston** or other small **butterhead lettuce**
2 **celery sticks**
½ **cucumber**
⅔ small **apple**
½ teaspoon **spirulina powder**
1 teaspoon **hemp seed oil**
ice cubes

Juice the kale with the spinach, lettuce, celery, cucumber, and apple. Stir in the spirulina powder and hemp seed oil.

Pour the juice into a glass over ice and serve immediately.

For healing beet juice, juice a generous ½ cup coarsely chopped kale with ½ cucumber, 2 beets, ⅔ small apple, and a ¾ inch piece peeled fresh ginger root. Stir in ½ teaspoon chlorella powder. Serve poured over ice.

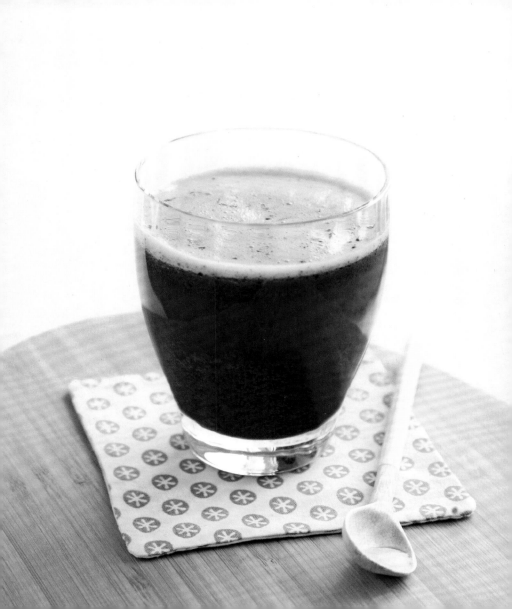

purple power juice

Makes **about 1¼ cups**
 (10 fl oz)

¾ inch piece fresh **ginger root**
1½ cups coarsely chopped
 red cabbage
1 **celery stick**
⅔ small **apple**
12 **red grapes**
ice cubes

Peel the ginger. Juice together the peeled ginger, cabbage, celery, apple, and grapes.

Pour the juice into a glass over ice and serve immediately.

For purple protein juice, juice 1½ cups coarsely chopped red cabbage with 12 red grapes, 1½ beets, and 4 large carrots. Whisk in 1 tablespoon protein powder and serve.

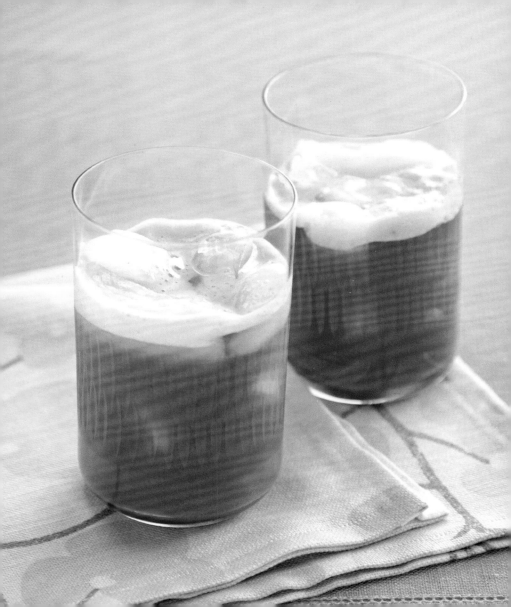

vitamin c punch

Makes **about 1 cup (8 fl oz)**

2 **lemons**
½ inch piece fresh **horseradish root**
⅔ small **apple**
¼ cup **parsley**

Coarsely peel the lemons. Juice all the ingredients together.

Pour the juice into a glass and serve immediately.

For spicy lemon tea, juice 2 coarsely peeled lemons and a ½ inch piece fresh horseradish root, pour into a cup, and fill with boiling water.

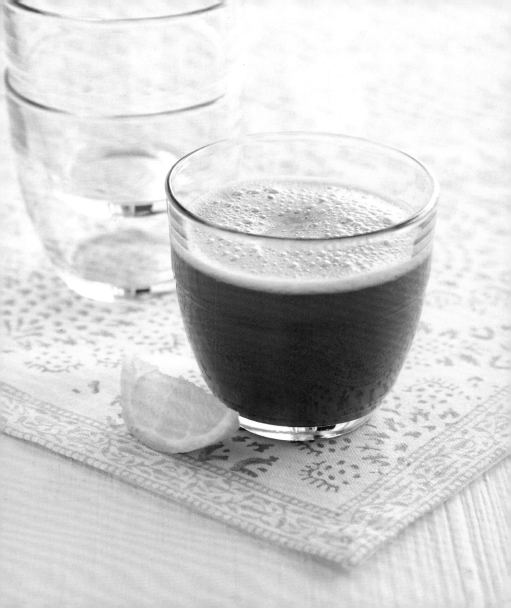

minty summer juice

Makes **about 1 ¼ cups**
  (10 fl oz)

6 **asparagus spears**
½ **cucumber**
4 small **carrots**
small handful of **mint**, plus an
  extra mint sprig to decorate
ice cubes

Juice together the asparagus, cucumber, carrots, and mint.

Pour the juice into a glass over ice, top with a sprig of mint, and serve immediately.

For spicy summer juice, juice 6 asparagus spears with ½ cucumber, ⅔ small apple, and a ¾ inch piece peeled fresh ginger root.

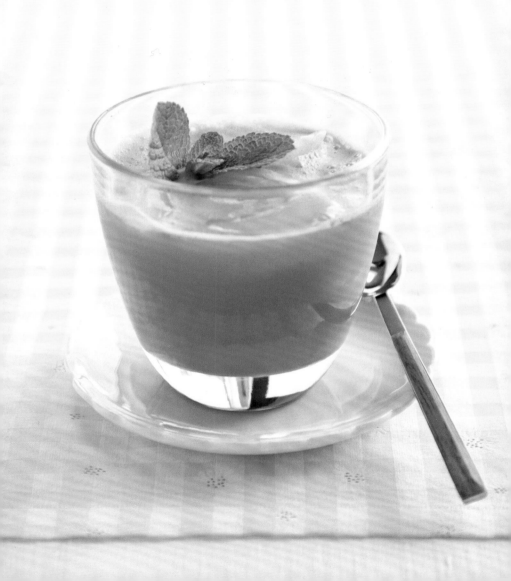

boost juice

Makes **about 1¾ cups (13½ fl oz)**

1 **pomegranate**
⅔ small **apple**
1½ **oranges**
5 **carrots**
1 cup **radish sprouts**

Remove the seeds from the pomegranate by cutting the fruit in half, then holding the halved fruit over a bowl and hitting the skin with a wooden spoon so that the seeds fall into the bowl. Juice all the ingredients together.

Pour the juice into a glass and serve immediately.

For spicy boost juice, juice 1½ oranges with ⅔ small apple, 5 carrots, 1 cup radish sprouts, and ½ red chile. Season with black pepper and serve.

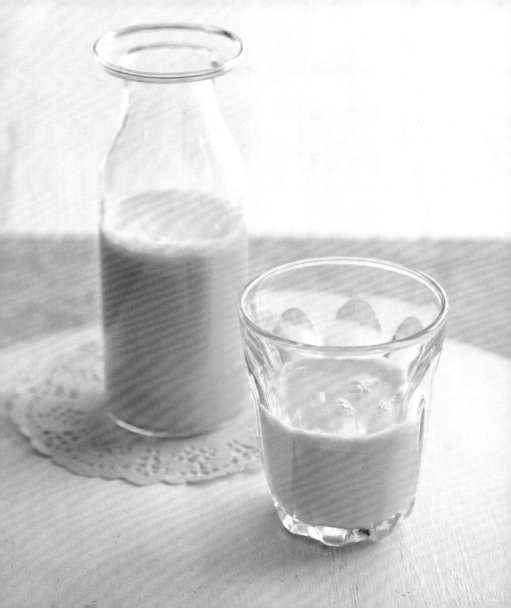

beet treat juice

Makes **about 1½ cups
(12 fl oz)**

⅛ **pineapple**, plus a pineapple
  wedge to decorate
1½ **oranges**
3½ **beets**
1½ cups coarsely chopped
  red cabbage

Coarsely peel the pineapple and the orange. Juice all the ingredients together.

Pour the juice into a glass, decorate with a wedge of pineapple, and serve immediately.

For sweet beet treat juice, juice 3½ beets with 3 oranges, ⅛ pineapple, coarsely peeled, and 2 peeled kiwifruit.

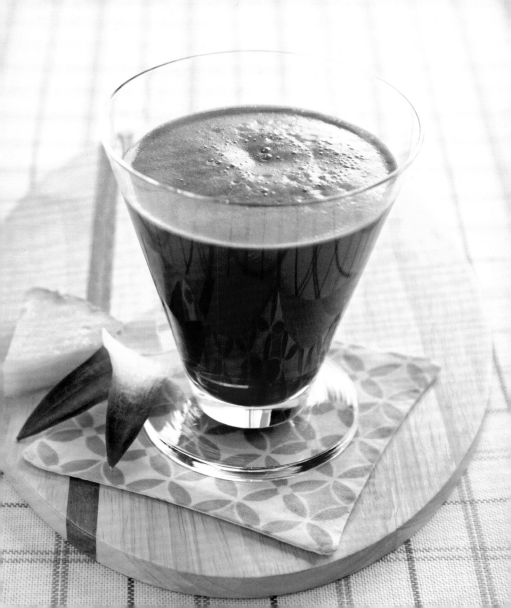

beautiful brussels juice

Makes **about 1¼ cups
(10 fl oz)**

¾ inch piece fresh **ginger root**
6 **Brussels sprouts**
2 **carrots**
⅔ small **apple**

Peel the ginger. Juice all the ingredients together.

Pour the juice into a glass and serve immediately.

For bountiful Brussels juice, juice 10 Brussels sprouts with 2 celery sticks, 2 carrots, 1 cup coarsely chopped broccoli, and ⅔ small apple.

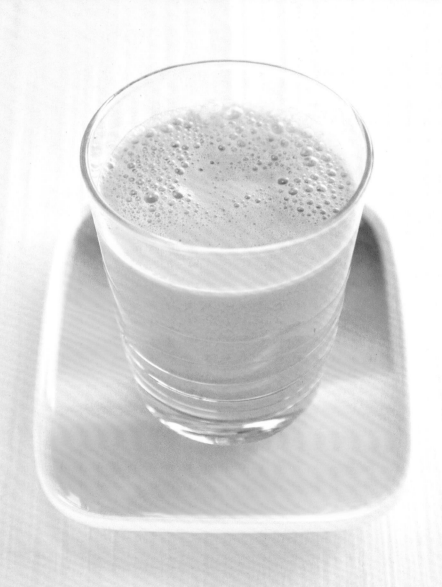

red refresher juice

Makes **about 1¼ cups
(10 fl oz)**

2 large **red bell peppers**
1 **lime**, plus extra to decorate
½ **cucumber**
1 cup coarsely chopped
   broccoli
ice cubes

Core and seed the bell peppers. Coarsely peel the lime. Juice together with the cucumber and broccoli.

Pour the juice into a glass over ice, add slices of lime, and serve immediately.

For red hot juice, core and seed 2 large red bell peppers. Juice the bell peppers with 1 small red chile, 4 large carrots, and 1⅓ cups coarsely chopped broccoli.

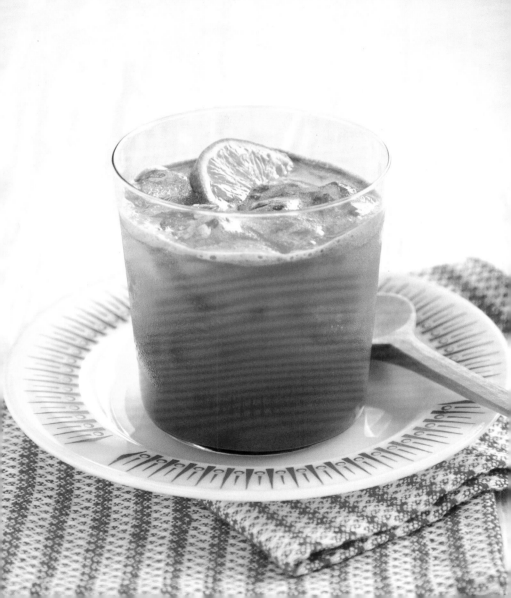

green goddess juice

Makes **about 1 ¼ cups (10 fl oz)**

¼ bunch of **broccoli**
2 **celery sticks**
1 large **apple**
¼ cup **cilantro leaves**
1–2 teaspoons **avocado oil**

Juice the broccoli with the celery, apple, and cilantro. Stir in the avocado oil.

Pour the juice into a glass and serve immediately.

For green refresher juice, juice ¼ bunch of broccoli with 2 celery sticks, 1 ⅓ cups watermelon chunks, and ½ cucumber. Serve poured over ice.

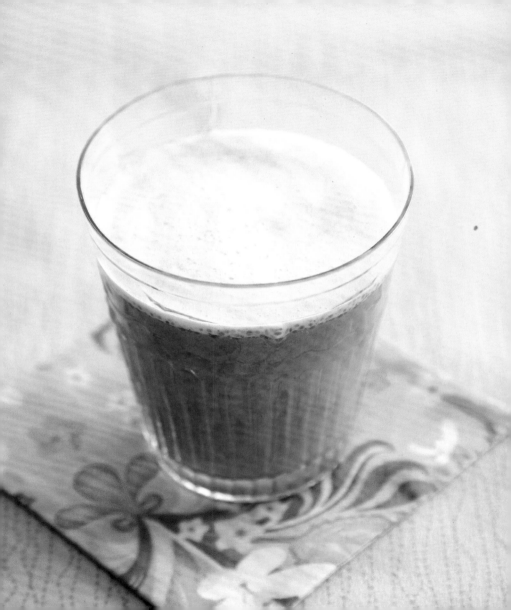

summer salad juice

Makes **about 1¼ cups (10 fl oz)**

1 **celery stick**
¼ **cucumber**
2 **tomatoes**
2 **Boston** or other small **butterhead lettuce**
4 large **carrots**
⅔ small **apple**
ice cubes

Juice together the celery, cucumber, tomatoes, lettuce, carrots, and apple.

Pour the juice into a glass over ice and serve immediately.

For minted summer salad juice, juice 1 romaine lettuce with ½ cucumber, 4 large carrots, ⅔ small apple, and a large bunch of mint. Serve poured over ice.

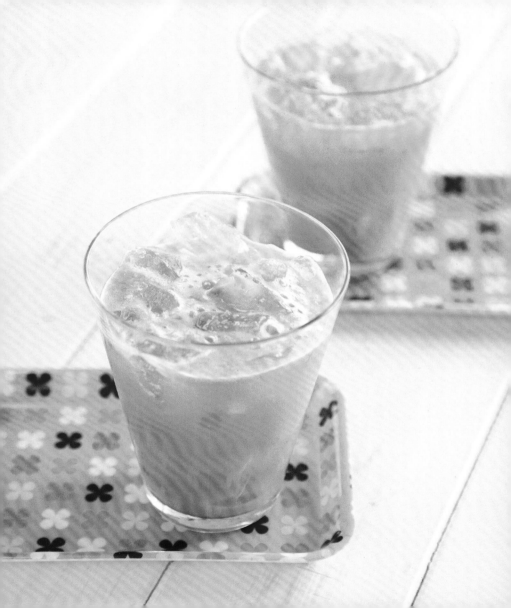

bell pepper punch

Makes **about 1¾ cups (13½ fl oz)**

1 large **red bell pepper**
1½ **beets**
4 large **carrots**
½ **lemon**
½ bunch of **watercress**
ice cubes
black pepper, to sprinkle

Core and seed the red bell pepper. Juice together with the beet, carrots, lemon, and watercress.

Pour the juice into a glass over ice, sprinkle with black pepper, and serve immediately.

For hot bell pepper punch, core and seed 1 large red bell pepper. Juice the bell pepper with 2 celery sticks, 3 tomatoes, 4 large carrots, and a ¾ inch piece fresh horseradish root.

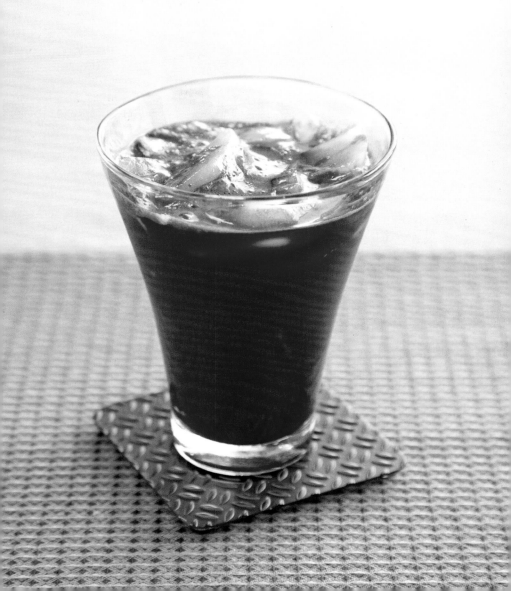

carrot, chile & pineapple juice

Makes about **scant 1 cup
(7 fl oz)**

½ small **chile**
¼ **pineapple**
4 **carrots**
ice cubes
juice of ½ **lime**
1 tablespoon chopped
cilantro leaves

Seed the chile. Remove the core and peel from the pineapple. Juice the carrots with the chile and pineapple.

Pour the juice into a glass over ice. Squeeze the lime juice over the top, stir in the chopped cilantro, and serve immediately.

For tomato, celery & ginger juice, trim 2½ celery sticks and peel and coarsely chop a 1 inch piece each of fresh ginger root and fresh horseradish root. Juice the celery, ginger, and horseradish with 3 tomatoes, 3 carrots, and a garlic clove. Serve over ice, decorated with celery slivers, if desired.

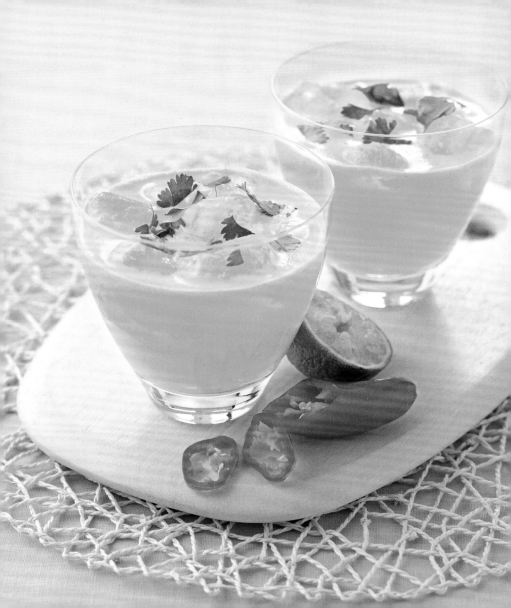

broccoli, spinach & apple juice

Makes **about scant 1 cup
(7 fl oz)**

¼ bunch of **broccoli**
5 cups **spinach**
1 **apple**
2–3 **ice cubes**

Trim the broccoli. Juice the apple with the spinach and broccoli, alternating the spinach leaves with the other ingredients so that the spinach leaves do not clog the machine.

Transfer the juice to a food processor or blender, add a couple of ice cubes, and process briefly.

Pour into a glass and serve immediately.

For spinach, apple & yellow pepper juice, use 1 large apple and, instead of broccoli, juice 1 yellow bell pepper. Stir in a pinch of ground cinnamon before serving.

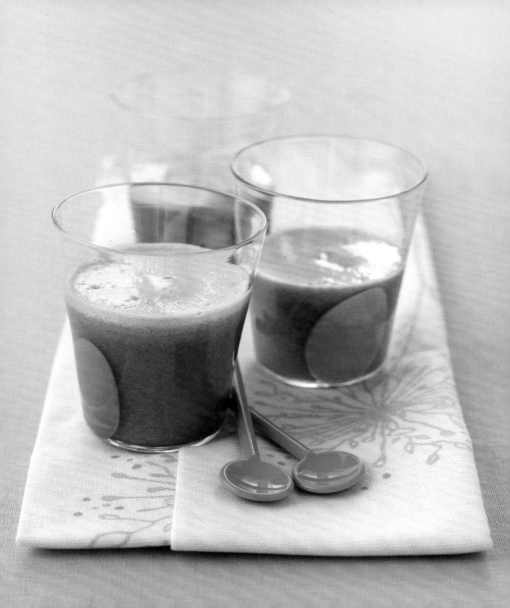

fennel & camomile juice

Makes about **1 cup**
(8 fl oz)

1 **lemon**, plus extra to
  decorate
²/₃ **fennel bulb**
½ cup chilled **camomile tea**
ice cubes

Coarsely peel the lemon and juice it with the fennel.
Mix the juice with the chilled camomile tea.

Pour the combined juice and tea into a glass over ice
and serve with slices of lemon to decorate.

For fennel & lettuce juice, juice ½ fennel bulb and
¼ head crisp lettuce with ½ lemon. Pour into a glass
over ice and decorate with a slice of lemon.

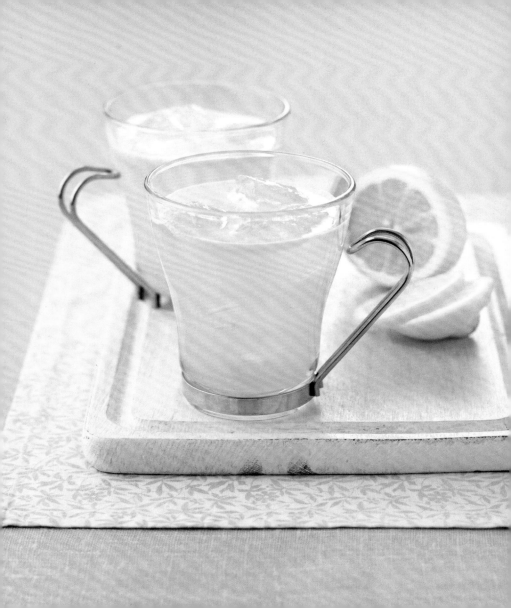

citrus detox juice

Makes **about 1¼ cups
(10 fl oz)**

2 **beets**
1½ **oranges**, coarsely peeled
3¼ cups coarsely chopped
   collard greens

Juice all the ingredients together.

Pour the juice into a glass and serve immediately.

For daily detox juice, juice 1 lemon with
1½ oranges and 3 cups coarsely chopped cabbage.
Stir in 1 teaspoon ground flaxseed and serve.

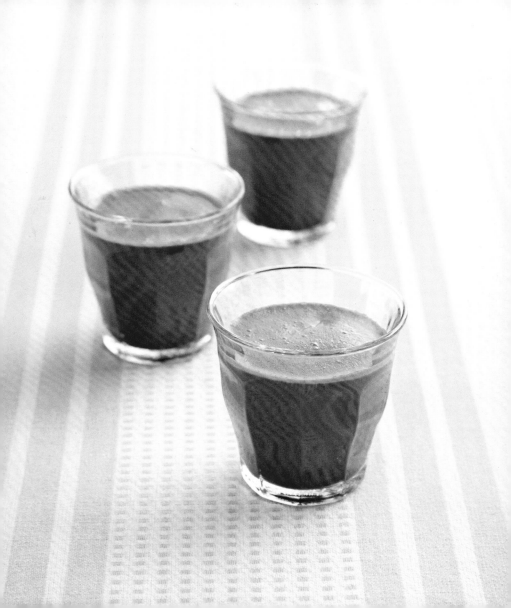

energy lift juice

Makes **about 1½ cups (12 fl oz)**

3 large **carrots**
2 **celery sticks**
1 large **sweet potato**
2¼ cups **spinach**

Juice all the ingredients together.

Pour the juice into a glass and serve immediately.

For fennel energy lift juice, replace the celery with 1 fennel bulb and juice as above. Serve sprinkled with a few fennel seeds.

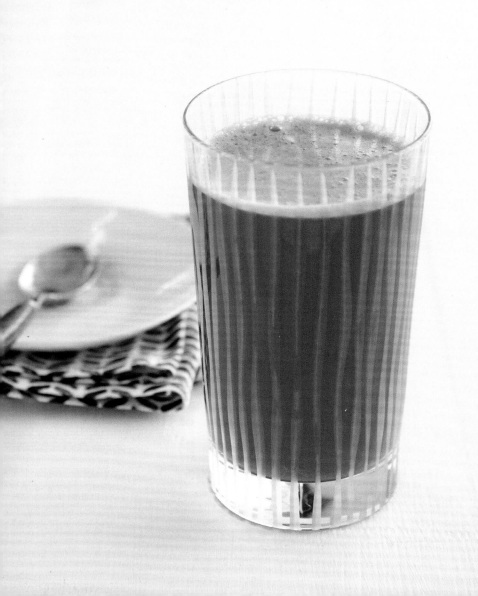

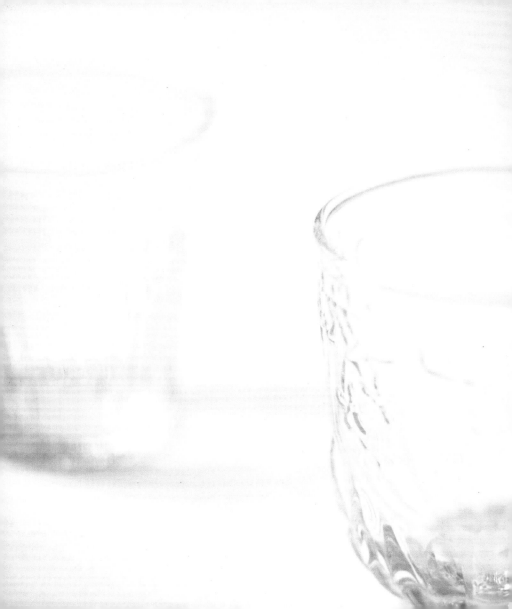

fruit juices

pear & cranberry juice

Makes about **1 cup (8 fl oz)**

1 pear
½ cup **cranberry juice**
ice cubes

Juice the pear, then mix the pear juice with the cranberry juice.

Pour the combined juices into a glass over ice and serve immediately.

For cranberry & cucumber juice, use the same amount of cranberry juice and add the juice of 1 orange and ⅙ cucumber.

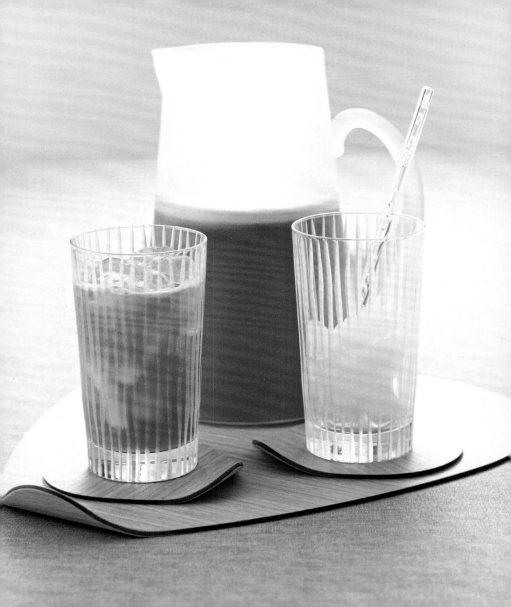

green lemonade

Makes **about 2 cups
(17 fl oz)**

2 **lemons**, plus extra
   to decorate
1 ¼ cups **spinach**
1 **cucumber**
sparkling water

Juice the lemons with the spinach and cucumber.

Pour the juice into a glass, fill with sparkling water, and decorate with a wedge of lemon.

For citrusade, replace the spinach with 2 ½ oranges and juice as above.

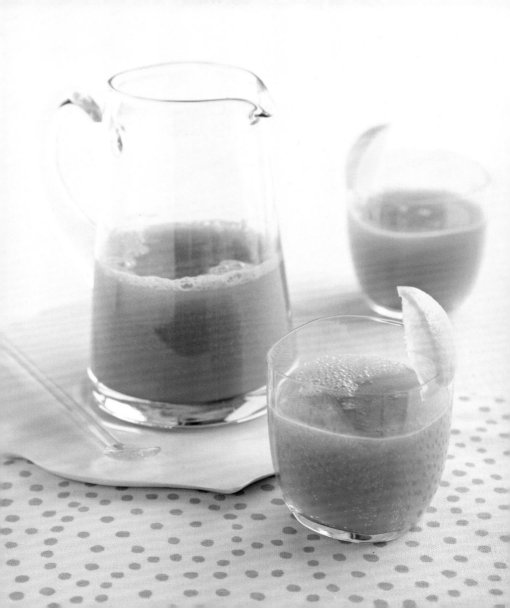

great grapefruit juice

Makes **about 1½ cups**
  (12 fl oz)

1 large **grapefruit**
1 large **kiwifruit**
²⁄₃ small **apple**, plus extra
  to decorate
½ **cucumber**

Coarsely peel the grapefruit and kiwifruit. Juice all the ingredients together.

Pour the juice into a glass, decorate with a slice of apple, and serve immediately.

For hot & spicy grapefruit juice, add a ¾ inch piece of peeled fresh ginger root to the other ingredients and juice as above.

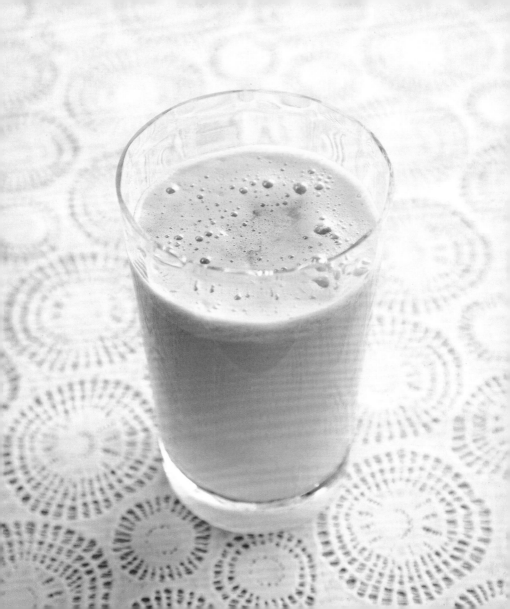

orange & raspberry juice

Makes about **2 cups**
  (17 fl oz)

3 **oranges**
1 ½ cups **raspberries**
1 cup **water**
ice cubes (optional)

Coarsely peel the oranges. Juice the oranges with the raspberries, then add the water.

Pour the juice into 2 tall glasses over ice, if using, and serve immediately.

For orange & apricot juice, juice 6 fresh, pitted apricots with 1 ½ oranges. Pour into tall glasses and fill with water to taste.

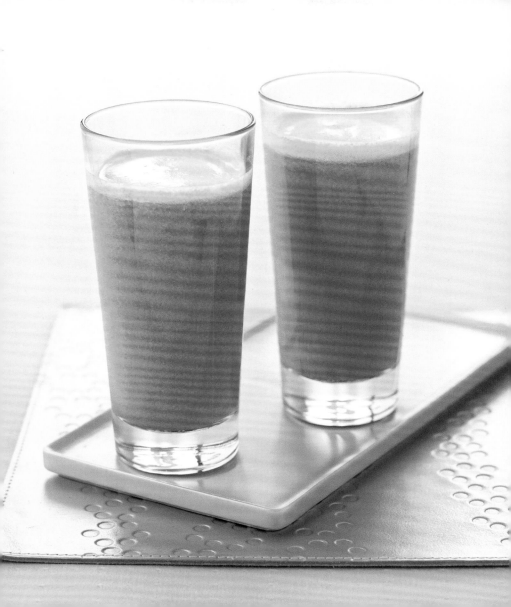

bouncing blueberry juice

Makes **about 1¼ cups (10 fl oz)**

2 cups **blueberries**
½ **cucumber**
⅔ small **apple**

Juice all the ingredients together.

Pour the juice into a glass and serve immediately.

For blueberry power juice, add 3 cups coarsely chopped red cabbage to the other ingredients and juice as above.

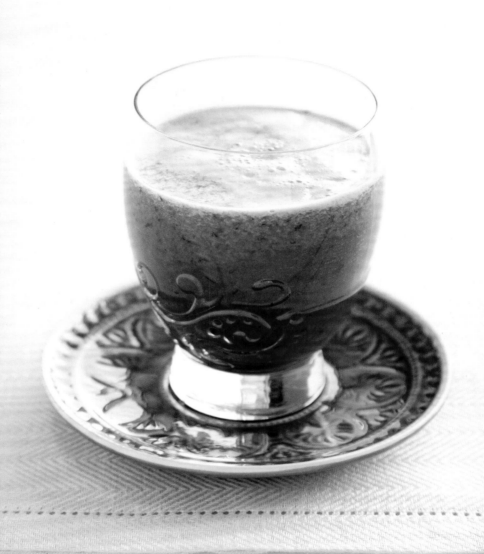

exotic elixir

Makes **about 1¼ cups
(10 fl oz)**

1½ **oranges**
1 large **kiwifruit**, plus extra
  to decorate
3 **apricots**
¼ **pineapple**
2 large **carrots**

Coarsely peel the orange and kiwifruit. Remove the pits from the apricots. Remove the skin from the pineapple. Juice all the ingredients together.

Pour the juice into a glass, decorate with a slice of kiwifruit, and serve immediately.

For exotic sparkling juice, juice the ingredients as above. Pour the juice into a tall glass over ice and serve filled with sparkling water.

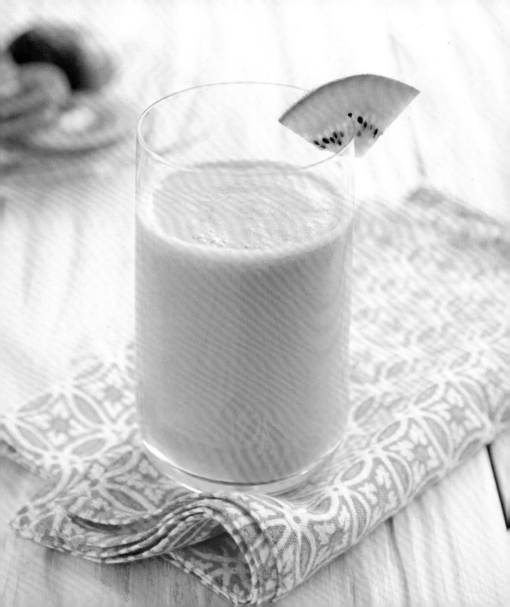

cool currants juice

Makes **about 1¼ cups
(10 fl oz)**

1 large **apple**
2 cups **black currants**
⅔ cup **red currants**
sprig of **black currants** or
   red currants, to decorate

Juice all the ingredients together.

Pour the juice into a glass, decorate with a sprig of currants, and serve immediately.

For currant & berry juice, replace ⅔ cup of the black currants with ⅔ cup mixed strawberries and blackberries and juice as above.

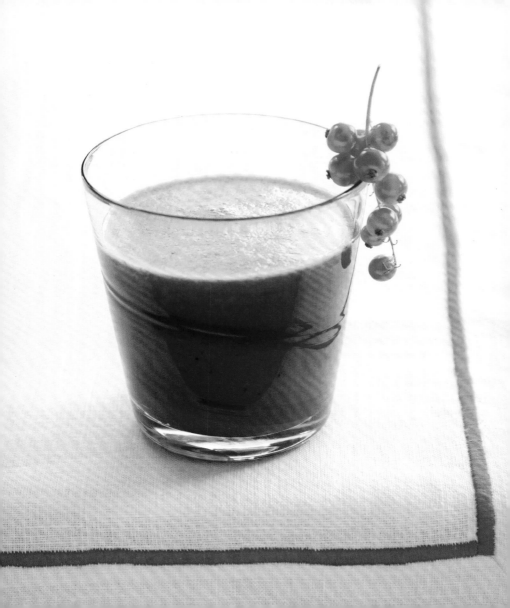

kiwi sparkler

Makes **about 1¼ cups
(10 fl oz)**

3 **kiwifruit**
¾ inch piece fresh
  ginger root
⅔ small **apple**
ice cubes (optional)
1¼ cups **sparkling water**

Peel the kiwifruit and ginger. Juice the kiwifruit with the ginger and apple.

Pour the juice into a tall glass over ice, if desired, fill with sparkling water, and serve immediately.

For apple & pear sparkler, juice 1 large apple with 2 small pears and a ¾ inch piece fresh ginger root. Pour into a tall glass and fill with sparkling water.

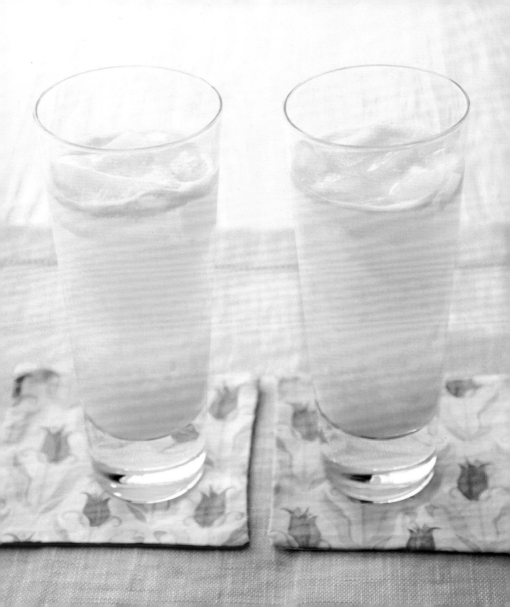

five fruits juice

Makes **about 1 ¼ cups (10 fl oz)**

3 **clementines**
6 **cherries**
1 ½ **apricots**
⅔ small **apple**
6 **red grapes**
1 **lemon grass** stalk
ice cubes

Peel the clementines. Pit the cherries and apricot. Juice together with the apple, grapes, and lemon grass.

Pour the juice into a glass over ice and serve immediately.

For five citrus juice, coarsely peel and juice 1 ½ clementines with 1 grapefruit, 1 ½ oranges, 1 lemon, and 1 lime. Serve poured over ice.

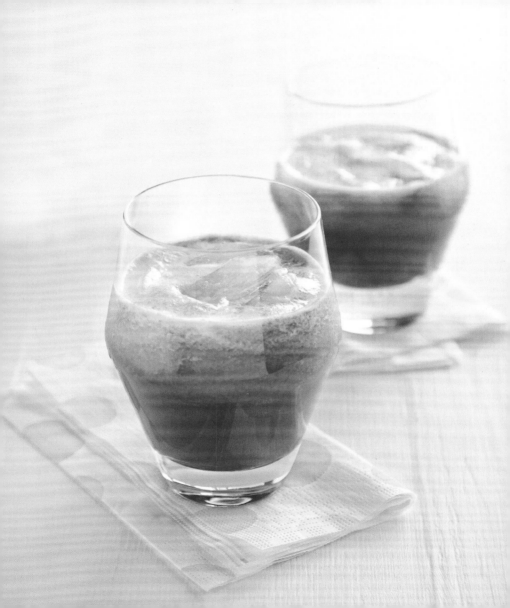

gingered pear juice

Makes **about 1 ¼ cups
(10 fl oz)**

¾ inch piece fresh
   ginger root
4 pears
large pinch of ground
   cinnamon
ice cubes

Peel the ginger. Juice the ginger with the pears. Stir in the cinnamon.

Pour the juice into a glass over ice and serve immediately.

For gingered mango juice, peel a ¾ inch piece fresh ginger root. Peel and pit 2 mangoes. Juice the ginger and mangoes with 1 large apple. Serve poured over ice.

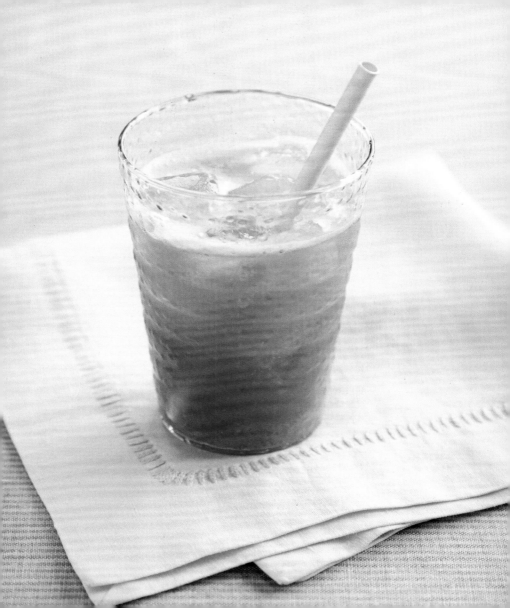

superfruits juice

Makes **about 1¼ cups
(10 fl oz)**

1 large **kiwifruit**
¼ cup fresh or frozen
  (defrosted) **cranberries**
¼ cup **pomegranate seeds**
⅔ cup **blueberries**
2 large **carrots**

Peel the kiwifruit. Juice all the ingredients together.

Pour the juice into a glass and serve immediately.

For superspicy juice, juice ¼ cup fresh or frozen (defrosted) cranberries with ¼ cup pomegranate seeds, a ¾ inch piece fresh ginger root, ⅔ small apple, and ¾ cup raspberries. Stir in a large pinch of grated nutmeg before serving.

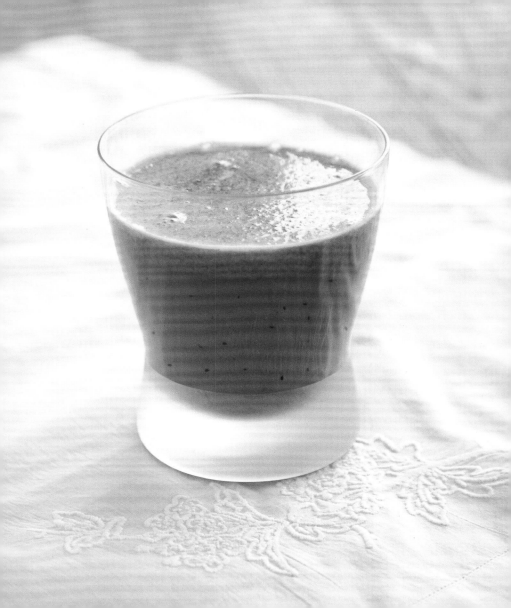

bitter berries juice

Makes **about 1¼ cups (10 fl oz)**

1½ cups coarsely chopped **green cabbage**
12 **strawberries**, plus extra to decorate
⅔ cup **blueberries**
¾ cup **raspberries**
8 **grapes**

Juice all the ingredients together.

Pour the juice into a glass, decorate with extra strawberries, and serve immediately.

For sweet berries juice, juice ⅔ cup each of strawberries, blackberries, raspberries, and blueberries with 3 carrots and a small handful of mint.

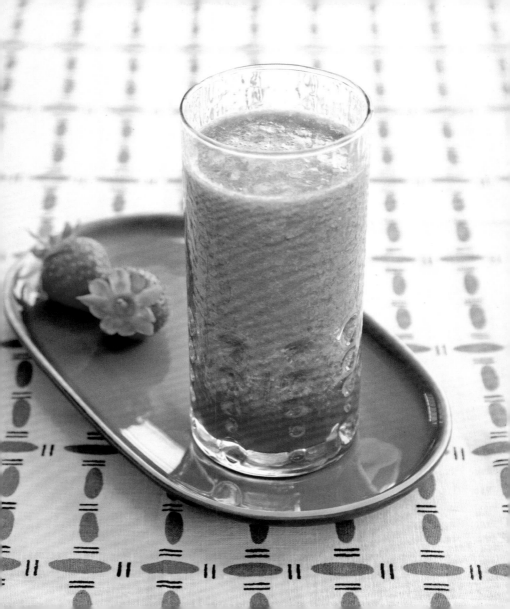

minty apple tea

Makes **about 2 cups
(17 fl oz)**

2 small **apples**
large handful **mint**, plus
extra sprigs to decorate
1 cup chilled **mint tea**
ice cubes

Juice the apples and mint. Stir in the chilled mint tea.

Pour the combined juice and tea into a glass over ice, decorate with a sprig of mint, and serve.

For cinnamon apple tea, juice 2 large apples. Stir in 1 cup chilled tea, add a large pinch of ground cinnamon, and stir to combine. Serve poured over crushed ice with a cinnamon stick for stirring.

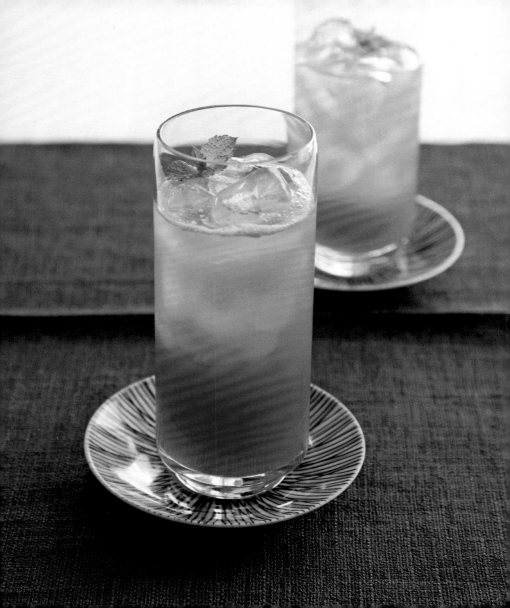

forest fruits juice

Makes **about 1¼ cups
(10 fl oz)**

1 ⅓ cups **blackberries**
⅔ cup **blueberries**
⅔ small **apple**

Juice all the ingredients together.

Pour the juice into a glass and serve immediately.

For green forest fruits juice, juice ⅔ small apple with 1 ⅓ cups blackberries, ½ cup coarsely chopped kale, and a ¾ inch piece peeled fresh ginger root.

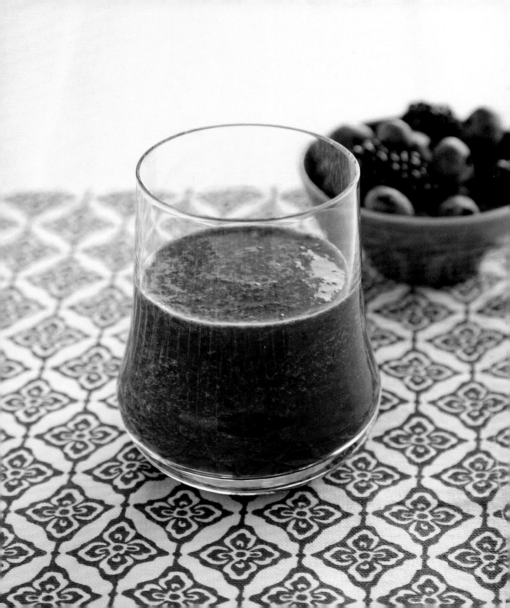

mango, melon & orange juice

Makes **about 1¾ cups
(13½ fl oz)**

3 **oranges**
1 ripe **mango**
¼ small **honeydew melon**
2 **ice cubes**

Coarsely peel and juice the oranges.

Pit and peel the mango, removing the melon as close to the skin as possible.

Put the mango and melon into a food processor or blender and process until smooth. Add the orange juice and ice cubes, then process until smooth.

Pour the juice into a glass and serve immediately.

For coconut & pineapple juice, put 1¾ cups coconut milk into a food processor or blender with ½ small pineapple, peeled, cored, and coarsely chopped. Process until smooth, then serve poured over ice and decorated with cherries or strawberries.

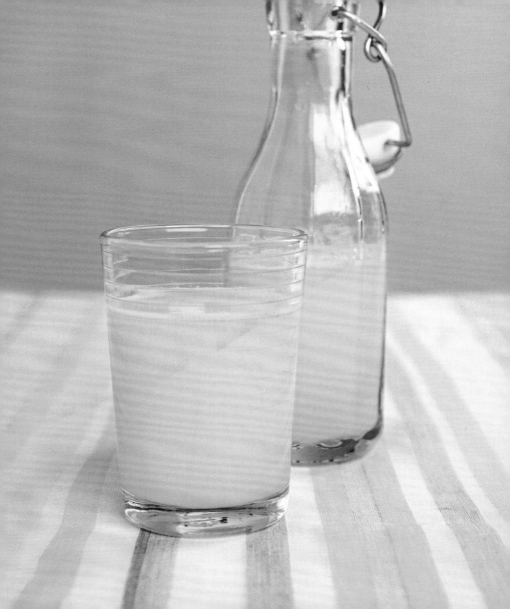

citrus green juice

Makes **about 1½ cups (12 fl oz)**

1 **lime**
1½ **oranges**
1 large **grapefruit**
1 teaspoon **agave syrup**
1½ teaspoons **wheatgrass powder**

Coarsely peel the lime, orange, and grapefruit. Juice all the fruits together. Stir in the agave syrup and wheatgrass powder.

Pour the juice into a glass and serve immediately.

For gingered green juice, juice 3 oranges with 4 large carrots, ⅔ small apple, and a ¾ inch piece peeled fresh ginger root. Stir in 1½ teaspoons barley grass or wheatgrass powder and serve.

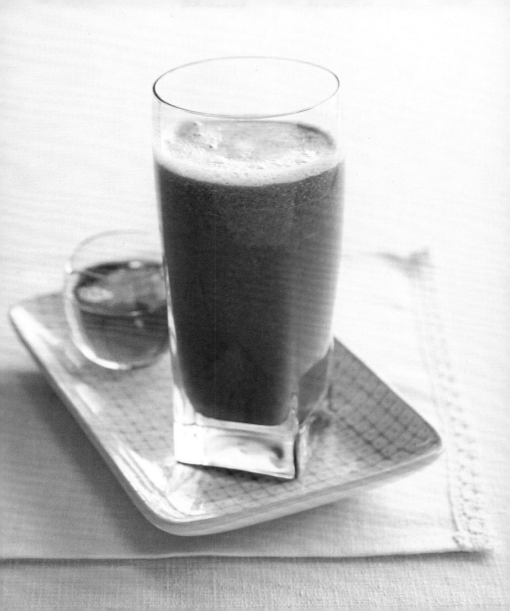

blackberry, melon & kiwifruit juice

Makes about **1 cup**
  (8 fl oz)

¼ small **cantaloupe melon**
2 **kiwifruit**
⅔ cup fresh or frozen
  blackberries, plus extra
  to decorate
2–3 **ice cubes**

Peel the melon as close to the skin as possible. Coarsely peel the kiwifruit. Juice the melon with the kiwifruit and blackberries.

Transfer the juice to a food processor or blender and process with a couple of ice cubes.

Pour into a glass and decorate with a few blackberries.

For melon & cherry juice, peel and coarsely chop ¼ honeydew melon. Juice the melon flesh with 1 cup pitted cherries and serve.

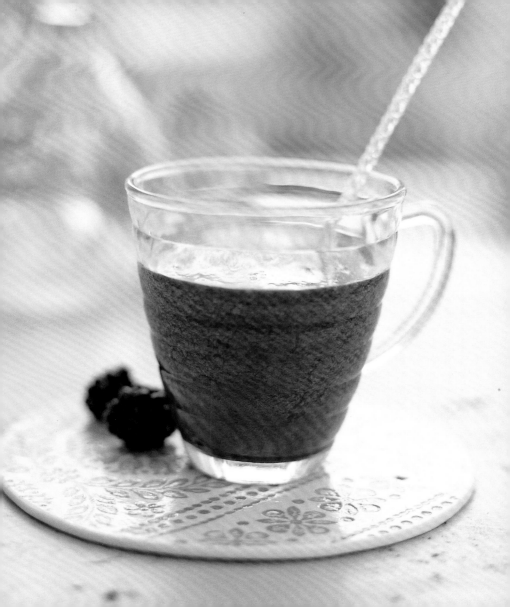

crazy cranberry juice

Makes **about 1½ cups
(12 fl oz)**

1½ **oranges**
2¼ cups **cranberries**
4 large **carrots**

Coarsely peel the orange. Juice the orange with the cranberries and carrots.

Pour the juice into a glass and serve immediately.

For cranberry fizz, juice 2¼ cups cranberries with ¾ cups raspberries and ⅔ small apple. Serve poured over ice and filled with sparkling water.

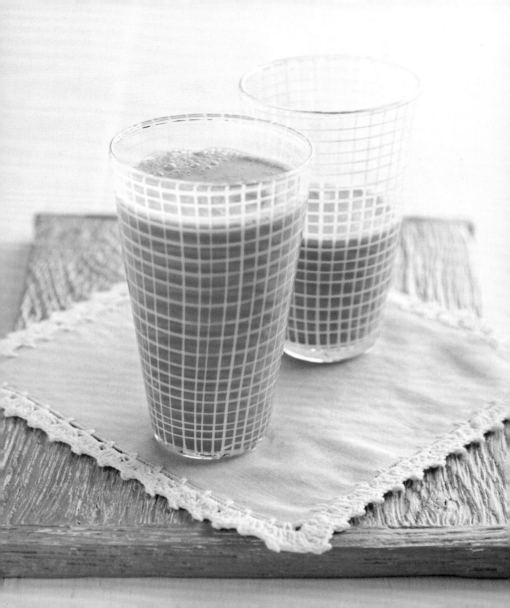

pineapple, grape & celery juice

Makes **about scant 1 cup**
  (7 fl oz)

⅛ **pineapple**
¾ cup **green grapes**
1 large **celery stick**
1 cup coarsely torn **lettuce**
2–3 **ice cubes** (optional)

Remove the skin and core from the pineapple. Juice the pineapple with the grapes, celery, and lettuce.

Pour the juice into a glass over ice, if using, and serve immediately.

For pineapple & pear juice, double the amount of pineapple and replace the grapes, celery, and lettuce with 2 pears and ½ a lime.

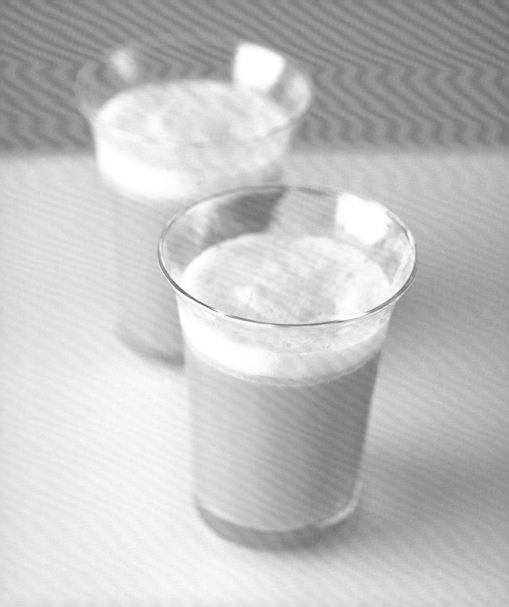

thick & creamy raspberry juice

Makes **about scant 1 cup (7 fl oz)**

1 large **apricot**
1⅔ cups **raspberries**,
   plus extra to decorate
12 **red grapes**
2 large **carrots**

Pit the apricot. Juice all the ingredients together.

Pour the juice into a glass, decorate with a few raspberries, and serve immediately.

For thick & creamy mango juice, pit 3 apricots. Peel and pit 1 mango. Juice the apricots and mango with 12 green grapes and 2 large carrots, and serve.

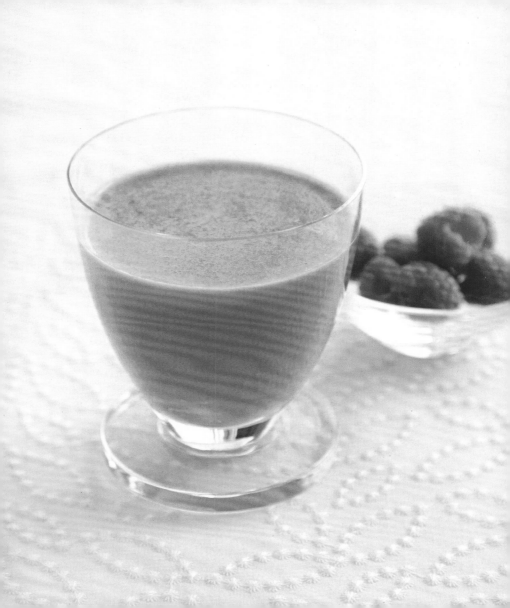

apple, cranberry & blueberry juice

Makes **about 1¼ cups
(10 fl oz)**

2 small **apples**
⅔ cup **unsweetened
cranberry juice**
1 cup fresh or frozen
blueberries
1 tablespoon **powdered
psyllium husks** (optional)
ice cubes (optional)

Juice the apples.

Transfer the apple juice to a food processor or blender,
add the cranberry juice, blueberries, and powdered
psyllium husks, if using, and process until smooth.

Pour the juice into a glass over ice, if using, and serve
immediately.

For cranberry, apple & lettuce juice, juice ⅓ small
apple and 2¼ cups coarsely torn lettuce with
½ cup cranberries. Serve over ice.

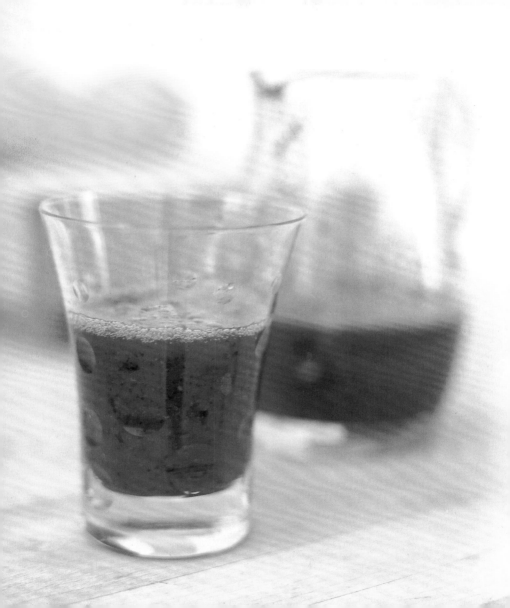

peachy plum juice

Makes **about 1 ¼ cups**
  (10 fl oz)

4 **plums**
3 **peaches**
3 **apricots**
2 large **carrots**
ice cubes

Remove the pits from the plums, peaches, and apricots. Juice all the ingredients together.

Pour the juice into a glass over ice and serve immediately.

For gingered plum juice, pit 4 plums. Juice the plums with 4 large carrots and a ¾ inch piece peeled fresh ginger root. Stir in a large pinch of grated nutmeg and serve.

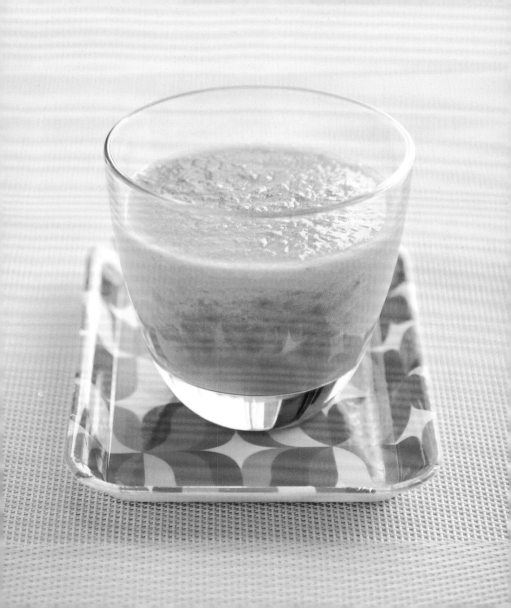

pomegranate plus juice

Makes **about 1 cup
(8 fl oz)**

1 **lemon**
2 **pomegranates**
1 ⅓ cups **blueberries**

Coarsely peel the lemon. Remove the seeds from the pomegranate by cutting the fruit in half, then holding the halved fruit over a bowl and hitting the skin with a wooden spoon so that the seeds fall into the bowl. Juice all the ingredients together.

Pour the juice into a glass and serve immediately.

For peachy pomegranate juice, remove the seeds from 1 pomegranate. Juice the pomegranate seeds with 2 pitted peaches, ⅔ small apple, and 2 large carrots.

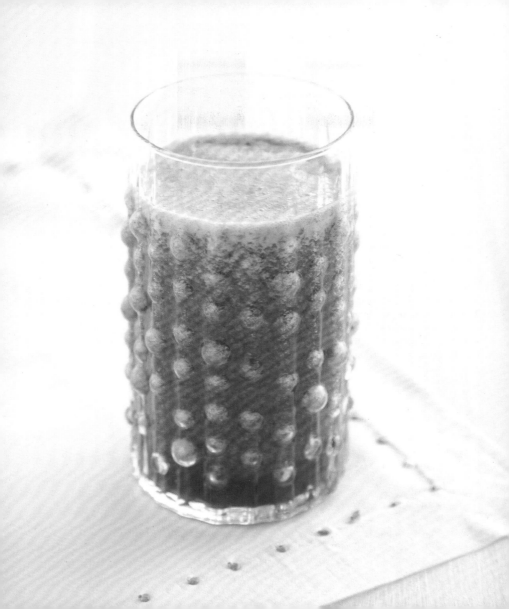

virgin pina colada juice

**Makes about 1¾ cups
(13½ fl oz)**

½ small **pineapple**, plus
  a small pineapple wedge
  to decorate
1 cup **coconut water**
ice cubes

Peel and juice the pineapple. Stir the coconut water into the pineapple juice.

Pour the combined juice and coconut water into a glass over ice, decorate with a wedge of pineapple, and serve immediately.

For mango & coconut juice, juice 2½ peeled and pitted mangoes. Stir in 1 cup coconut water and serve poured over ice with a slice of mango to decorate.

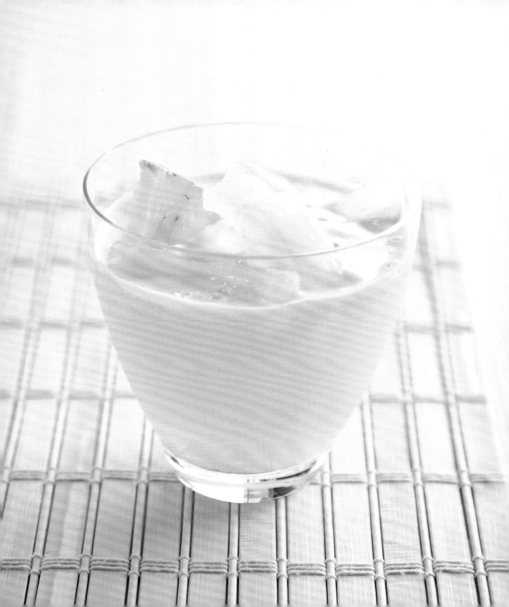

blackberry, apple & celeriac juice

Makes about **scant 1 cup
(7 fl oz)**

¼ **celeriac (celery root)**
¼ large **apple**
⅔ cup frozen **blackberries**,
 plus extra to decorate
2–3 **ice cubes**

Peel the celeriac. Juice the celeriac with the apple.

Transfer the juice to a food processor or blender, add
the blackberries and the ice cubes, and process briefly.

Pour the juice into a glass, decorate with extra
blackberries, and serve immediately.

For blackberry & pineapple juice, juice 1 cup each of
blackberries and pineapple chunks with ⅛ apple. Serve
in a tall glass over ice.

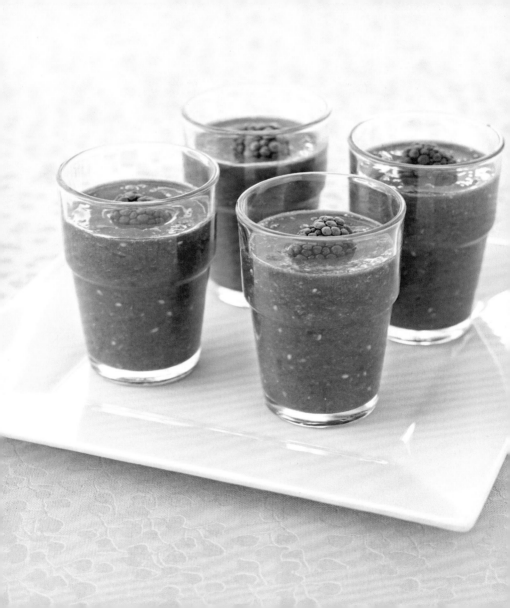

watermelon & raspberry juice

Makes **about scant 1 cup
(7 fl oz)**

10 oz **watermelon**
  (2 cups prepared)
1 cup **raspberries**
crushed ice (optional)

Peel the melon as close to the skin as possible and coarsely chop.

Transfer the watermelon and raspberries to a food processor or blender and process until smooth.

Press the juice through a strainer over a bowl to remove any raspberry seeds.

Pour the juice into glasses over some crushed ice, if desired.

For melon & apple juice, put 1 1/3 cups peeled and chopped honeydew melon into a food processor or blender with 2/3 small green apple, cored and cut into wedges. Add 1 tablespoon lemon juice and process until smooth. Pour over crushed ice, if desired.

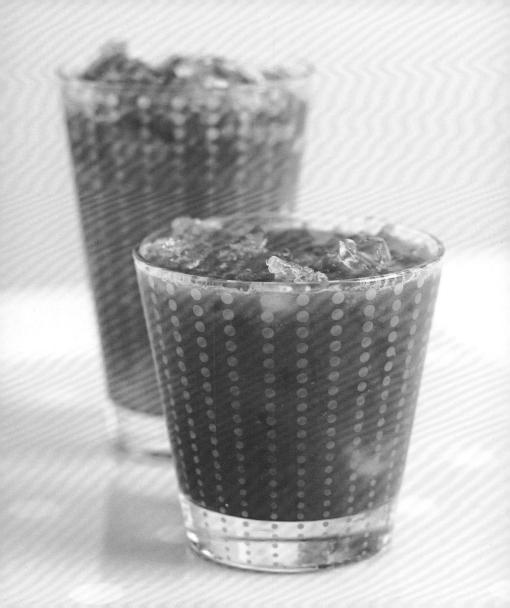

pear, kiwifruit & lime juice

Makes **about 1¼ cups (10 fl oz)**

3 **kiwifruit**, plus extra to decorate
2 **pears**
½ **lime**
2–3 **ice cubes** (optional)

Peel the kiwifruit. Juice the kiwifruit with the pears and lime.

Pour into a tall glass, add the ice cubes, if using, decorate with slices of kiwifruit, and serve immediately.

For grape & kiwifruit juice, replace the pears and lime with 2 cups green grapes.

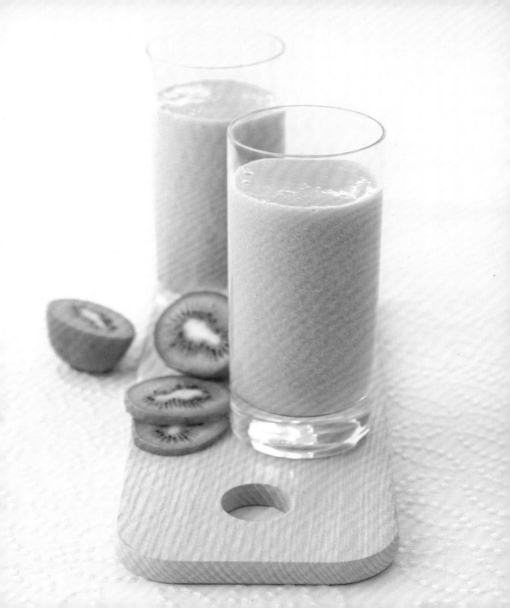

spiced melon juice

Makes **about scant 2 cups
(15 fl oz)**

½ **cantaloupe**
⅛ **watermelon**
2 cups **spinach**
¾ inch piece fresh **ginger root**
2–3 **ice cubes**
grated **nutmeg**, to sprinkle

Peel both melons as close to the skin as possible. Juice the melons with the spinach and ginger.

Transfer the juice to a food processor or blender, add a handful of ice cubes, and process for 10 seconds.

Serve in a glass, sprinkled with nutmeg.

For spicy melon & carrot juice, replace the spinach with 2 large carrots and juice as above.

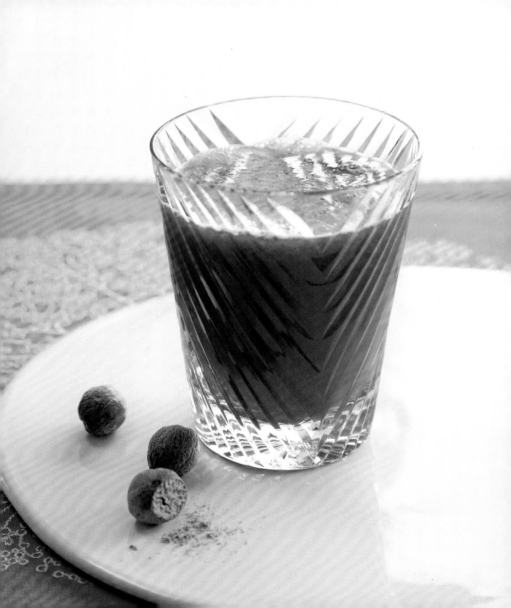

juicy
smoothies

banana & maple syrup smoothie

Serves **2**

2 bananas
1 ¼ cups **milk**
¼ cup **plain fromage blanc**
  or **Greek yogurt**
3 tablespoons **maple syrup**
¼ cup hot **oatmeal**

To decorate
banana slices
raisin bread chunks

Peel and chop the bananas.

Put the bananas into a food processor or blender with the milk, fromage blanc or Greek yogurt, and maple syrup and process until smooth. Add the oatmeal and process again to thicken.

Pour into 2 glasses. Arrange banana slices and chunks of raisin bread on 2 toothpicks and balance them across the top of the glasses to decorate.

For peanut butter smoothies, replace the bananas with ¼ cup chunky peanut butter, and change the maple syrup to honey. Make as above, processing until smooth.

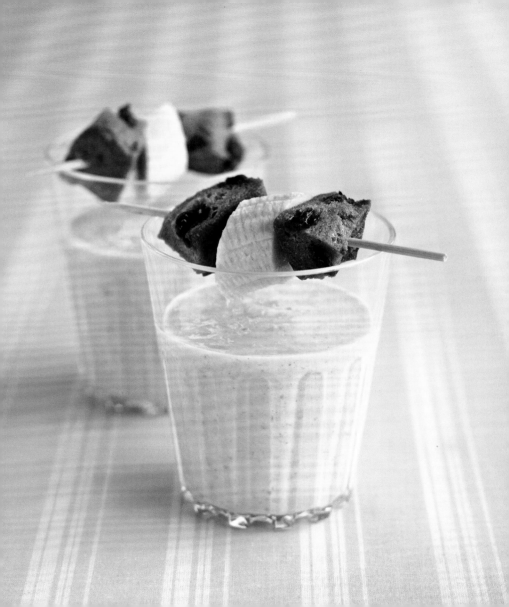

breakfast smoothie

Serves **2**

3 **oranges**
1 **banana**
2 tablespoons **muesli**
1¼ cups **milk**
ground **cinnamon**, to sprinkle

Coarsely peel and juice the oranges. Peel the banana.

Transfer the orange juice and banana to a food processor or blender, add the muesli and milk, and process until smooth.

Pour the smoothie into 2 glasses, sprinkle with ground cinnamon, and serve immediately.

For nutty breakfast smoothie, follow the recipe above, replacing 1 tablespoon muesli with 1 tablespoon nuts of your choice (walnuts and pecans both work really well).

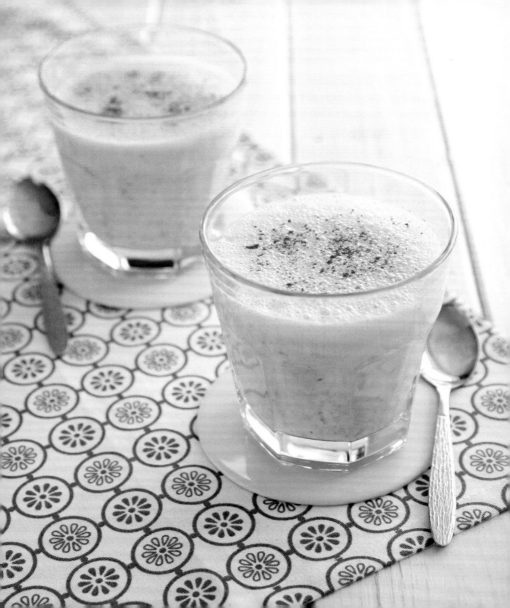

shocking pink smoothie

Serves **2**

1 ½ **beets**
1 **banana**
½ cup hulled **strawberries**,
  plus extra to decorate
½ cup **raspberries**
1 tablespoon **slivered
  almonds**
1 ¼ cups **milk**
ice cubes

Juice the beets. Peel the banana.

Transfer the beet juice and banana to a food processor or blender, add the berries, almonds, and milk, and process until smooth.

Pour the smoothie into 2 tall glasses over ice, decorate with strawberries, and serve immediately.

For shocking pink protein boost, follow the recipe above, adding 2 tablespoons whey protein powder to the food processor or blender with the other ingredients. If the smoothie is a little too thick, just add another dash of milk.

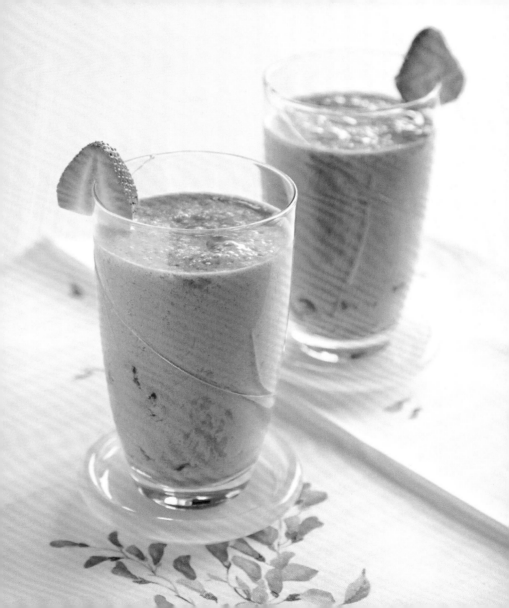

digestive delight smoothie

Serves **2**

1 **papaya**
2 **apricots**
1 **lime**, plus extra to decorate
1¾ cups **hemp milk**
1 teaspoon **chia oil**
¼ teaspoon ground **cinnamon**

Peel and seed the papaya. Pit the apricot. Coarsely peel and then juice the lime.

Transfer the papaya, apricot, and lime juice to a food processor or blender, add the remaining ingredients, and process until smooth.

Pour the smoothie into 2 glasses, add a wedge of lime to each glass, and serve immediately.

For minty digestive delight smoothie, follow the recipe above, adding 10–12 mint leaves to the food processor or blender with the other ingredients.

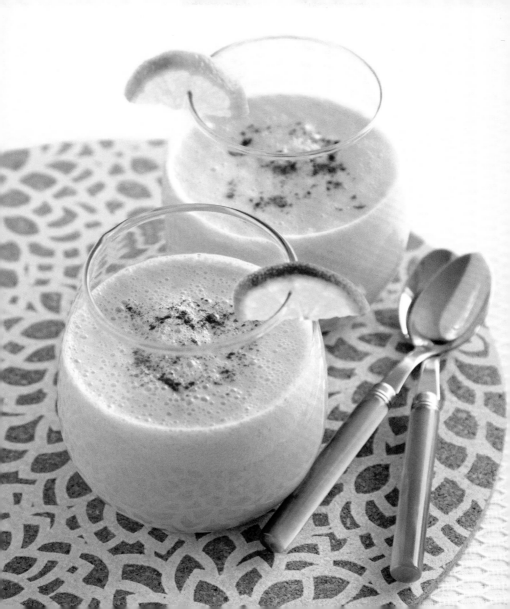

strawberries & custard smoothie

Serves **1**

1½ **oranges**
1 **mango**
½ cup **milk**
½ cup hulled **strawberries**

Coarsely peel and then juice the oranges. Pit and peel the mango.

Transfer the orange juice and mango to a food processor or blender, add the milk, and process until smooth. Pour the mixture into a glass.

Put the strawberries into the food processor or blender with 1 tablespoon of water and process until smooth.

Pour the strawberry mixture into the glass on top of the mango mixture. Stir a little to create swirls of the strawberry mixture in the smoothie.

For raspberries & custard smoothie, follow the recipe above, replacing the strawberries with ¾ cup raspberries.

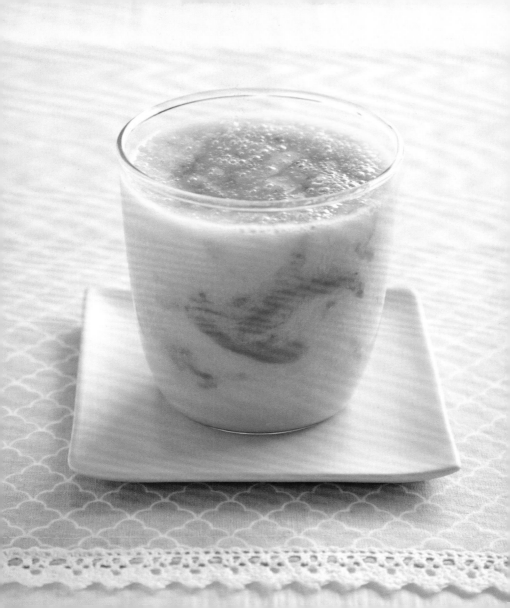

perfect passion smoothie

Serves **4**

1 **lime**
2 large **mangoes**
5 **passionfruit**
1 cup **plain yogurt**
2 handfuls **ice cubes**

Coarsely peel and then juice the lime. Peel and pit the mangoes.

Transfer the lime juice and mangoes to a food processor or blender. Halve the passionfruit, scoop out the pulp, and add all but 1 tablespoon to the blender with the yogurt and ice cubes and process until smooth.

Pour the smoothie into 4 glasses, decorate with the remaining passionfruit pulp, and serve immediately.

For passionfruit & banana smoothie, juice 1 coarsely peeled lime. Transfer the juice to a food processor or blender, add 2 peeled bananas, the pulp of 4 passionfruit, and 2½ cups milk, and process until smooth.

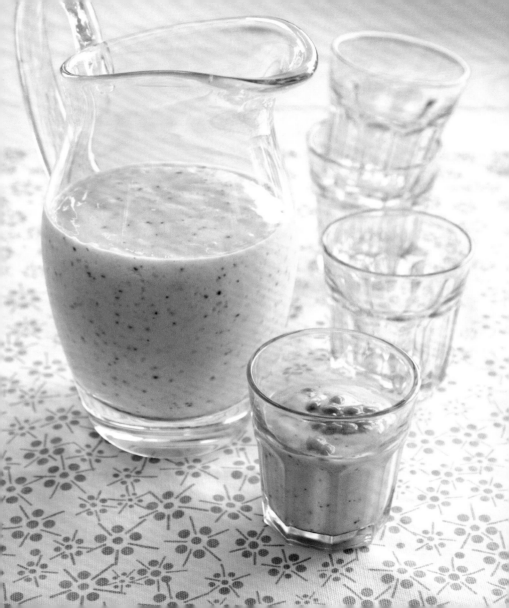

nectarine & raspberry yogurt ice

Serves **2**

3 **nectarines**
1½ cups **raspberries**
⅔ cup **plain yogurt**
handful of **ice cubes**

Halve and pit the nectarines.

Put the nectarines and raspberries into a food processor or blender and process until really smooth. Add the yogurt and process again, then add the ice and process until crushed and the shake thickens.

Pour into 2 chilled glasses. Decorate with cocktail umbrellas, if desired.

For banana & mango coconut ice, replace the nectarines and raspberries with 1 large banana and 1 mango, peeled, pitted, and cut into chunks, and process until smooth. Add ⅔ cup coconut milk and process again. Add the ice and process until the shake thickens. Pour into chilled glasses to serve.

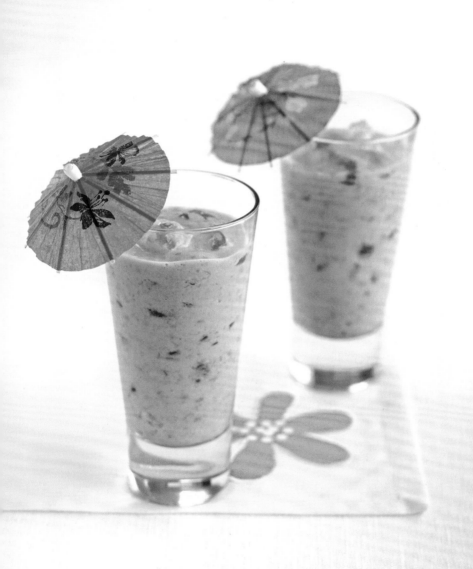

probiotic smoothie

Serves **1**

1½ **oranges**
1 **mango**
¾ cup **kefir** or **plain
probiotic yogurt**
1 cup **blueberries**

Coarsely peel and then juice the orange. Peel and pit the mango.

Transfer the orange juice and mango to a food processor or blender, add the kefir or yogurt and blueberries, and process until smooth.

Pour the smoothie into a glass and serve immediately.

For kefir & berry smoothie, juice 1½ coarsely peeled oranges. Transfer the juice to a food processor or blender, add 1 cup kefir or plain probiotic yogurt and 1 cup frozen mixed berries, and process until smooth.

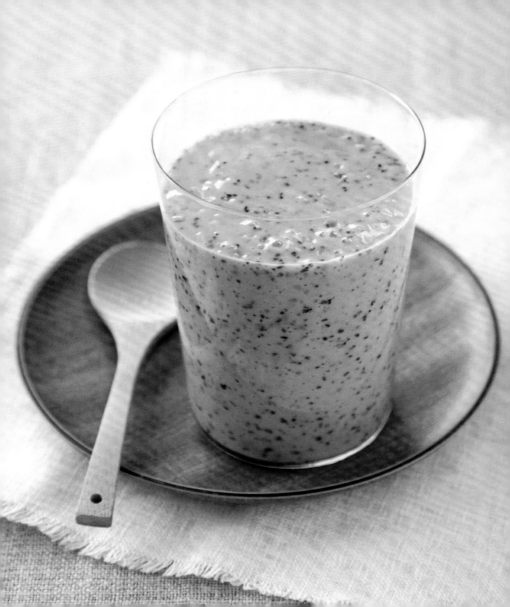

energizer smoothie

Serves **2**

2½ **beets**
6 pitted **dates**
1 tablespoon **rolled oats**
⅔ cup **blackberries**
1 teaspoon **maca powder**
2 cups **almond milk**
1 teaspoon **ground flaxseed**
ice cubes

Juice the beets.

Transfer the juice to a food processor or blender, add the remaining ingredients (except the ice cubes), and process until smooth.

Pour the smoothie into 2 glasses over ice and serve immediately.

For spicy energizer smoothie, juice 2½ beets with a 1¼ inch piece peeled fresh ginger root and 1 lemon grass stalk. Transfer the juice to a blender or food processor, add 6 figs, 1 tablespoon rolled oats, ⅔ cup hulled strawberries, 1 teaspoon maca powder, and 2 cups almond milk, and process until smooth.

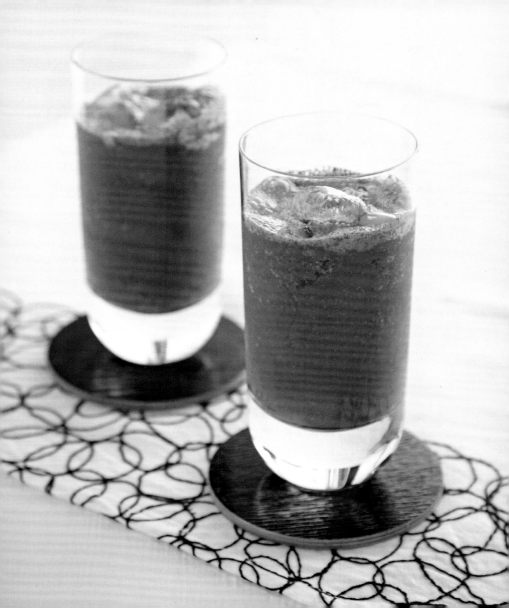

superfood smoothie

Serves **2**

¼ cup **cranberries**
⅓ cup **pomegranate seeds**
⅓ cup coarsely chopped **kale**
1 large **beet**
1 **banana**
1 tablespoon **goji berries**
⅓ cup **strawberries**
2 cups **hemp milk**
1 tablespoon **avocado oil**
1 tablespoon **toasted sesame seeds**, to sprinkle

Juice the cranberries with the pomegranate seeds, kale, and beet.

Transfer the juice to a food processor or blender, add the remaining ingredients, and process until smooth.

Pour the smoothie into 2 glasses, sprinkle with toasted sesame seeds, and serve immediately.

For superfood green smoothie, juice ¾ cup coarsely chopped kale with 2 celery sticks and a ¾ inch piece peeled fresh ginger root. Transfer the juice to a food processor or blender, add 1 peeled and pitted avocado, 1 peeled garlic clove, 1 cucumber, ¼ cup parsley, salt and black pepper, and a large handful of ice cubes, and process until smooth.

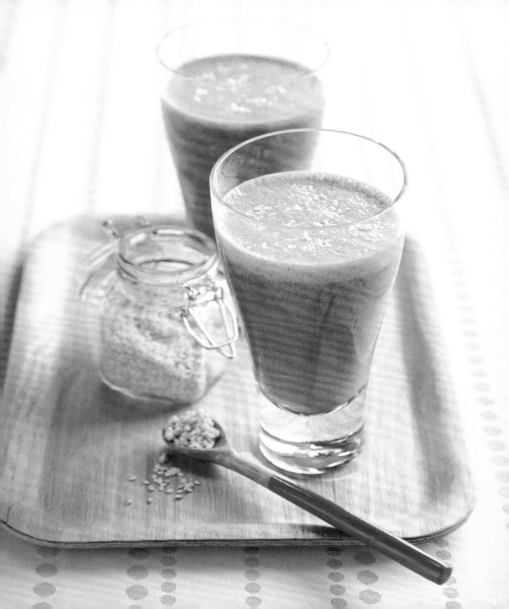

berry blast smoothie

Serves **2**

1 large **apple**
1 large **banana**
2 cups **mixed berries** (such
   as blueberries, blackberries,
   raspberries, and hulled
   strawberries), plus
   extra to decorate
ice cubes

Juice the apple. Peel the banana.

Transfer the apple juice and banana to a food processor or blender, add the mixed berries, and process until smooth, adding a little water, if necessary, if you want a looser consistency.

Pour the smoothie into 2 glasses over ice, decorate with a few extra berries, and serve immediately.

For berry green smoothie, follow the recipe above, adding 2¼ cups spinach to the juicer with the apple.

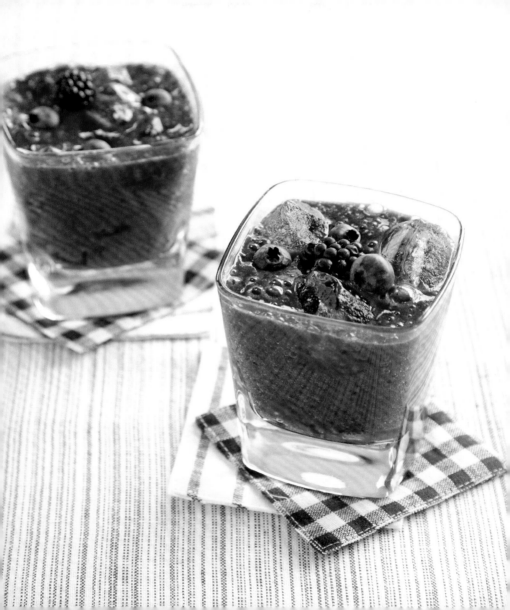

cherry & chocolate smoothie

Serves **2**

²⁄₃ cup **blueberries**
1 ½ cups **cherries**
1 tablespoon **cocoa nibs,**
  plus extra to sprinkle
1 ¼ cups **milk**

Juice the blueberries. Pit the cherries.

Transfer the blueberry juice and cherries to a food processor or blender, add the cocoa nibs and milk, and process until smooth.

Pour the smoothie into 2 glasses, sprinkle with some extra cocoa nibs, and serve immediately.

For breakfast cherry & chocolate smoothie, follow the recipe above, adding 1 tablespoon cashew nuts and 1 tablespoon rolled oats to the food processor or blender with the other ingredients.

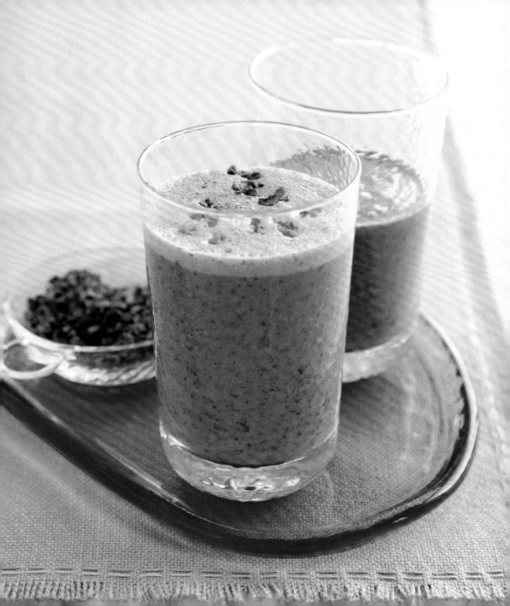

peanut butter & banana smoothie

Serves **4**

½ **lime**
1 large **banana**
1 tablespoon **peanut butter**
1¼ cups **almond milk**
grated **nutmeg**, to sprinkle

Coarsely peel and then juice the lime. Peel the banana.

Transfer the lime juice and banana to a food processor or blender, add the peanut butter and almond milk, and process until smooth.

Pour the smoothie into 4 glasses, sprinkle with a large pinch of nutmeg, and serve immediately.

For peanut butter & blueberry smoothie,
coarsely peel and juice ½ lime. Transfer the juice to a food processor or blender, add ⅔ cup blueberries, 1 tablespoon peanut butter, and 1¼ cups milk, and process until smooth.

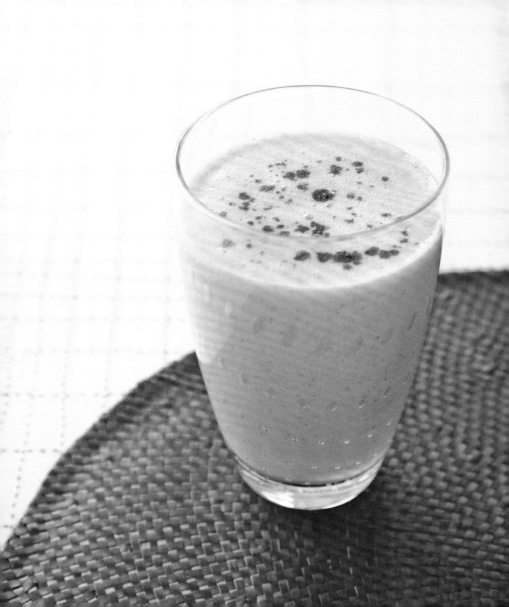

fruity summer shake

Serves **4**

2 **peaches**
2 cups hulled **strawberries**
2½ cups **raspberries**
1¾ cups **milk**
ice cubes

Halve and pit the peaches.

Put the peaches into a food processor or blender with the strawberries and raspberries and process to a smooth puree. Add the milk and blend the ingredients again until the mixture is smooth and frothy.

Pour the shake into 4 tall glasses over the ice cubes.

For soy milk & mango shake, replace the peach, strawberries, and raspberries with 2 large mangoes, peeled and pitted, and the juice of 2 oranges. Puree as above, then pour in 1¾ cups soy milk, blend, and serve over ice cubes as above.

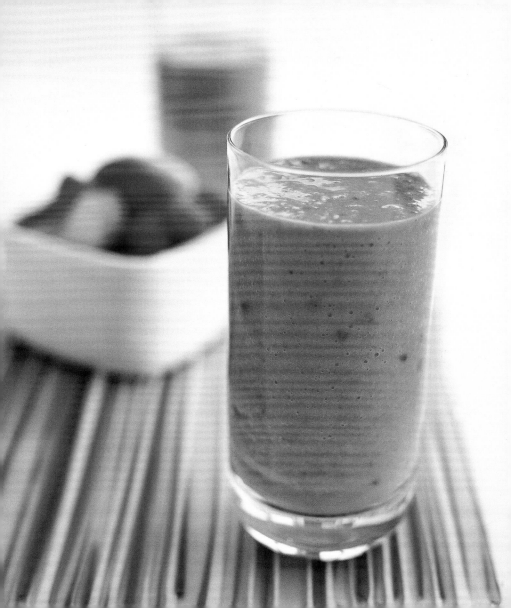

bursting baobab smoothie

Serves **4**

1 large **orange**
1 **mango**
1 small **banana**
3 **ice cubes**
1 tablespoon **baobab powder**
(available online)
1¼ cups **water**

Coarsely peel and then juice the orange. Peel and pit the mango. Peel the banana.

Transfer the orange juice to a food processor or blender, add the mango, banana, and the remaining ingredients, and process until smooth.

Pour the smoothie into glasses and serve immediately.

For bursting blueberry smoothie, juice 1 large beet. Transfer the juice to a food processor or blender, add 1 small peeled banana, 1½ cups blueberries, 3 ice cubes, 1 tablespoon baobab powder, and 1¼ cups water, and process until smooth.

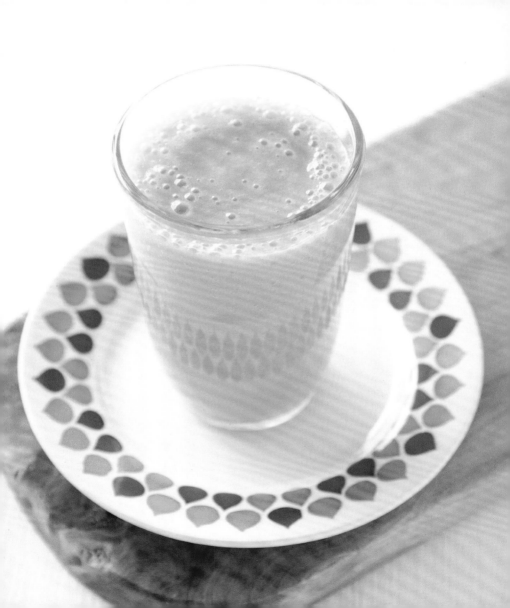

extra-thick berry smoothie

Serves **4**

3 tablespoons **crème de cassis** or **spiced red fruit syrup**

2 cups **mixed frozen berries**

2 cups fat-free **fromage blanc** or **Greek yogurt**

1¾ cups **milk**

1 **vanilla bean**, split in half lengthwise

toasted slivered almonds, to decorate

Put the crème de cassis or syrup into a saucepan over low heat and gently heat, then add the berries. Stir, cover, and cook for about 5 minutes or until the fruit has thawed and is beginning to collapse. Remove from the heat and cool completely.

Process most of the berry mixture with the fromage blanc or yogurt and milk in a food processor or blender until smooth.

Scrape in the seeds from the vanilla bean and beat to combine.

Fold the reserved berries into the fromage blanc mixture until just combined. Spoon into 4 glasses and serve immediately, decorated with toasted almonds.

For extra-thick exotic fruit smoothie, replace the crème de cassis with 3 tablespoons coconut milk and the mixed berries with 2 cups coarsely chopped exotic fruits, such as mango and pineapple, and add 1 tablespoon lime juice. Heat as above, then blend in a food processor or blender until smooth. Chill as above. Mix the fromage blanc or Greek yogurt with 2 tablespoons coconut milk and 1¾ cups milk. Fold in the fruit puree and serve sprinkled with toasted coconut flakes, if liked.

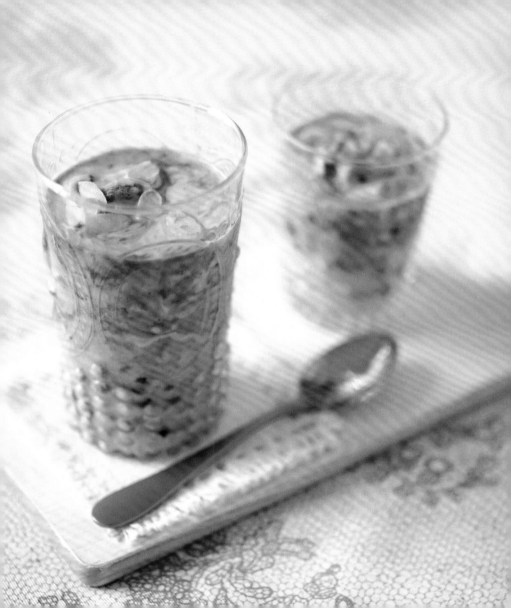

recovery smoothie

Serves **4**

2 **kiwifruit**
5 **dried figs**
1¼ cups **almond milk**
1 tablespoon **protein powder**
4 **walnut halves**
¼ teaspoon ground
   cinnamon

Peel and then juice the kiwifruit.

Transfer the juice to a food processor or blender, add the remaining ingredients, and process until smooth.

Pour the smoothie into 4 glasses and serve immediately.

For nutty recovery smoothie, peel and juice 2 kiwifruit. Transfer the juice to a food processor or blender, add 3 tablespoons peanut butter, 1¼ cups almond milk, 1 tablespoon cocoa nibs, and 1 tablespoon protein powder, and process until smooth.

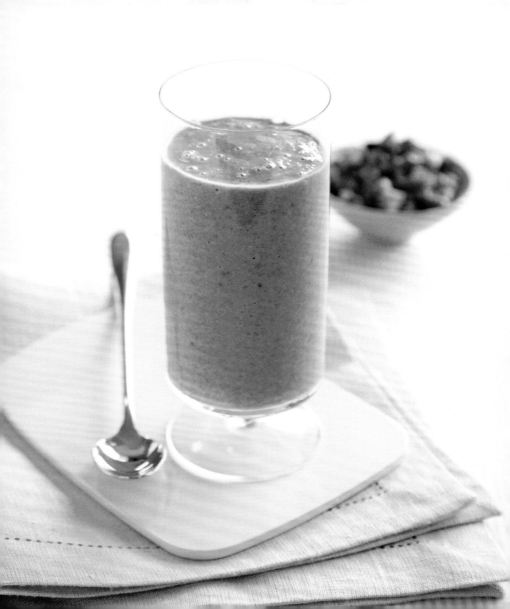

creamy green smoothie

Serves **2**

1 **avocado**
1 **lime**
1 ¼ cups **spinach**
2 **celery sticks**, plus extra
  to decorate
1 **garlic clove**
½ cup **parsley**
1 teaspoon **green powder**
  (such as spirulina,
  wheatgrass or chlorella)
salt and **black pepper**

Peel and pit the avocado. Coarsely peel the lime. Juice the lime with the spinach.

Transfer the avocado and the juice to a food processor or blender, add the remaining ingredients and enough water to just cover, and process until smooth. Season the smoothie to taste with salt and black pepper and process again.

Pour the smoothie into 2 glasses, add a trimmed celery stick to each glass, and serve immediately.

For spicy green smoothie, follow the recipe above, adding a ¾ inch piece peeled fresh ginger root and ½ seeded red chile to the food processor or blender with the other ingredients.

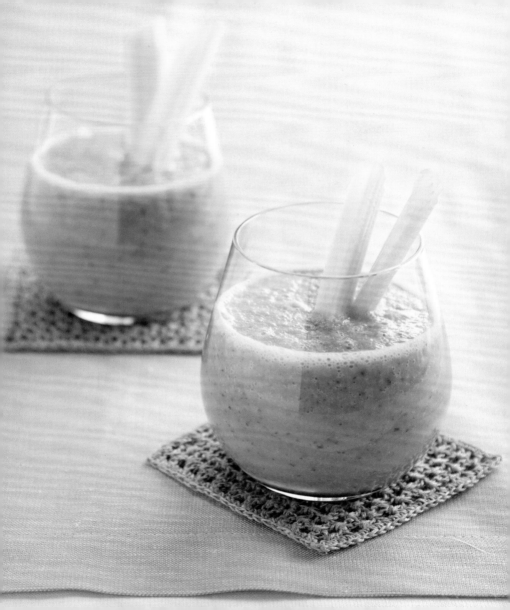

melon, mint & berry smoothie

Serves **4**

¼ **watermelon** (about 2 lb)
14–16 **strawberries**
12 **mint leaves**
small handful of **ice cubes**

Peel the melon as close to the skin as possible. Hull the strawberries.

Put all the ingredients into a food processor or blender and process until smooth.

Pour into 4 glasses and serve immediately.

For melon, mint & strawberry soup, put 1⅓ cups peeled, seeded, and chopped cantaloupe into a food processor or blender and process until smooth. Pour into a pitcher, cover, and chill for 20 minutes. Clean the food processor or blender and repeat with 1 small peeled, seeded, and chopped honeydew melon and then 1 cup hulled and chopped strawberries. When ready to serve, pour a ladle of each fruit puree into a bowl and make a pattern by dragging a knife through each one. Serve sprinkled with 2 tablespoons hulled and chopped strawberries and 2 teaspoons chopped mint.

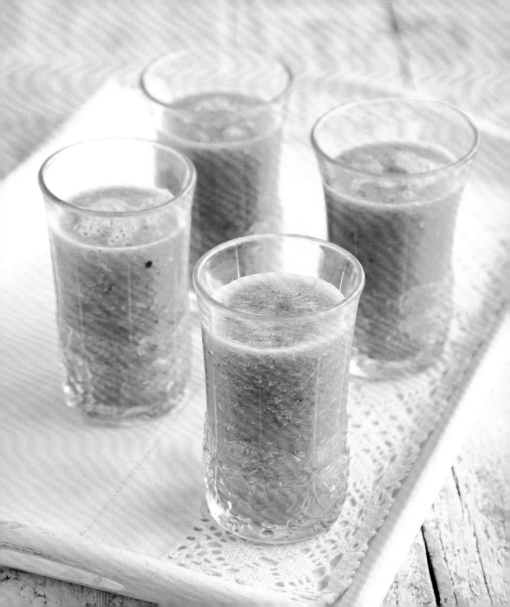

summer smoothie

Serves **1**

½ **lime**
small handful **mint**, plus
  an extra sprig to decorate
¾ cup **gooseberries**
⅓ cup **ground almonds**
⅔ cup **nondairy milk**
1 teaspoon **elderflower
  cordial** or **syrup**
  (available online)

Coarsely peel the lime. Juice the lime with the mint.

Transfer the juice to a food processor or blender, add the remaining ingredients, and process until smooth.

Pour the smoothie into a glass, decorate with a sprig of mint, and serve immediately.

For strawberry summer smoothie, juice ½ coarsely peeled lime and a small handful of mint. Transfer the juice to a food processor or blender, add ¾ cup hulled strawberries, ⅓ cup ground almonds, and ⅔ cup milk, and process until smooth. Decorate with a sprig of mint.

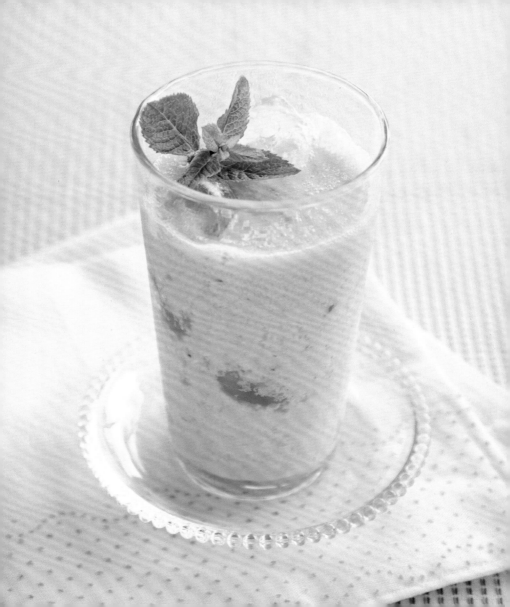

mango & passion fruit smoothie

Serves **4**

1 large **mango**
3 cups **plain yogurt**
1–2 tablespoons **agave nectar**, to taste
1 **vanilla bean**, split in half lengthwise
4 **passionfruit**, halved

Pit and peel the mango.

Transfer the mango to a food processor or blender and process to a puree.

Put the yogurt and agave nectar, according to taste, into a large bowl, scrape in the seeds from the vanilla bean, and beat together. Gently fold in the mango puree and spoon into tall glasses.

Scoop the seeds from the passion fruit and spoon over the smoothie. Serve immediately with thin cookies, if desired.

For black currant & almond smoothie, puree 1¾ cups black currants as above and fold into the yogurt with the agave nectar, according to taste, and 1 teaspoon almond extract. Spoon into tall glasses and decorate with toasted almonds to serve.

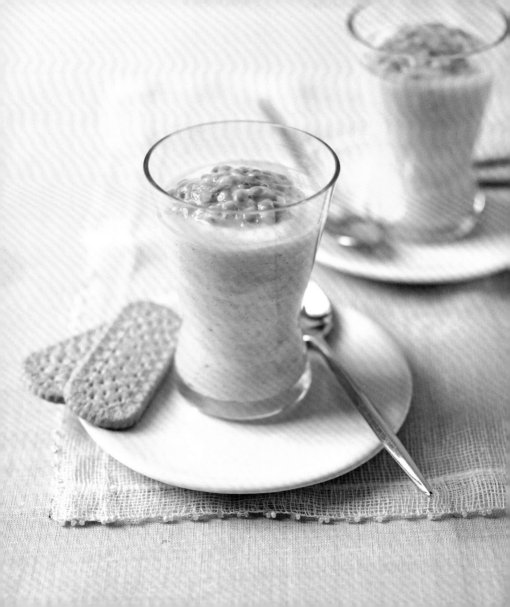

blueberry & mint smoothie

Serves **2**

⅔ cup **frozen blueberries**
⅔ cup **soy milk**
small bunch of **mint**

Put the blueberries into a food processor or blender and pour in the soy milk. Pull the mint leaves off their stems, reserving one or two sprigs for decoration, and add the remainder to the blender. Process briefly.

Pour the smoothie into 2 glasses, decorate with the reserved mint sprigs, and serve immediately.

For blueberry & apple smoothie, process 2 apples with 1 cup blueberries in a food processor or blender until smooth.

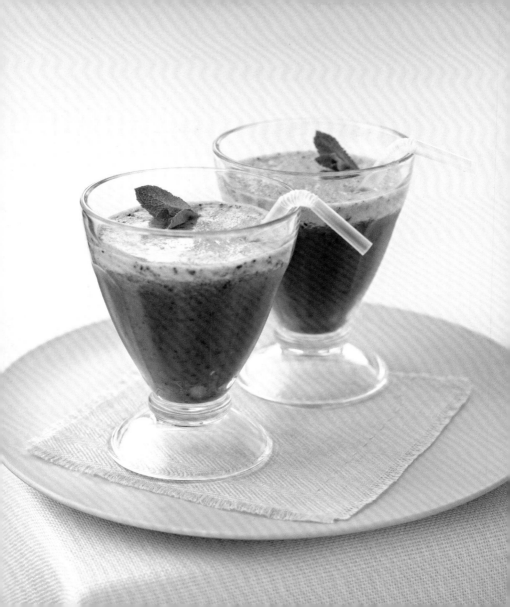

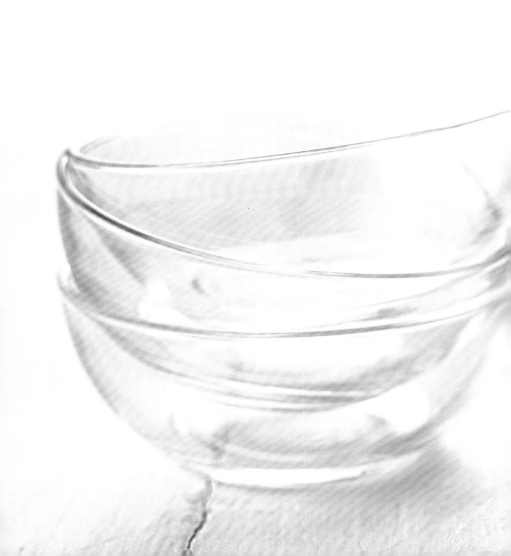

juicy dips

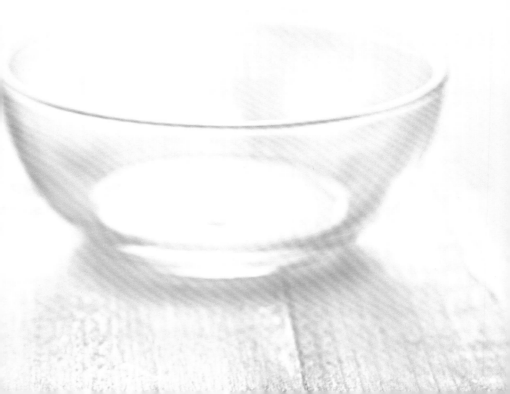

red pepper & scallion dip

Serves **4**

1 large **red bell pepper**,
   cut into quarters, cored,
   and seeded
2 **garlic cloves,** unpeeled
1 cup **plain yogurt**
2 **scallions**, finely chopped
black pepper
selection of **raw vegetables**,
   such as carrots, cucumber,
   bell peppers, fennel bulb,
   tomatoes, baby corn, snow
   peas, celery, and zucchini,
   cut into batons, to serve

Slightly flatten the bell pepper quarters and put onto a baking sheet. Wrap the garlic in aluminum foil and put onto the sheet. Roast in a preheated oven, at 425°F, for 30–40 minutes, until the bell pepper is slightly charred and the garlic is soft.

When cool enough to handle, remove the skin from the bell pepper and discard. Transfer the flesh to a food processor or blender. Squeeze in the roasted garlic flesh from the cloves and process until smooth.

Stir in the yogurt and scallions. Season to taste with black pepper and serve with the vegetable batons.

For eggplant & yogurt dip, roast a whole eggplant in a preheated oven, at 425°F, with the garlic for 30–40 minutes, omitting the red bell pepper. If the eggplant is still not tender after the cooking time, carefully turn it over and bake for another 10–15 minutes, until soft. Cut the eggplant in half and scoop out the flesh into a food processor or blender. Squeeze in the roasted garlic flesh from the cloves, add a handful of basil, and season with salt and black pepper. Process until smooth. Stir in the yogurt and scallions. Serve with the vegetable batons.

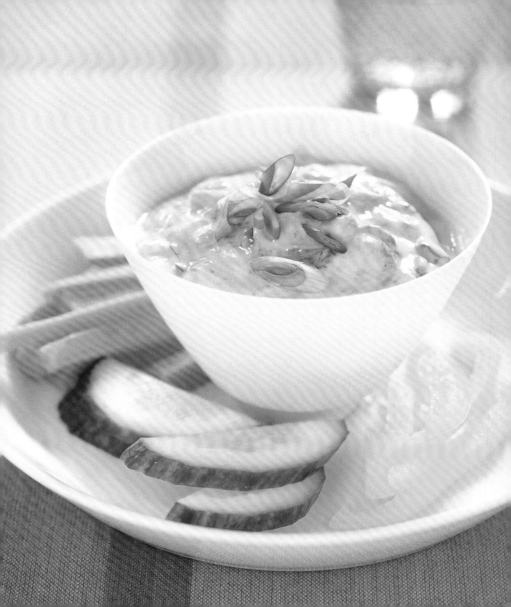

spinach & bean dip

Serves **2**

2 cups **baby spinach**
1 **celery stick**
1 (15 oz) can **cannellini
(white kidney) beans**,
drained
salt and **black pepper**
vegetable crudités, to serve

Juice the spinach with the celery.

Pour the juice into a food processor or blender, add the cannellini beans, and process until smooth. Season to taste and serve with vegetable crudités.

For nutty bean dip, follow the recipe above, adding ½ cup walnuts (or your favorite nuts) to the food processor or blender with the juice and kidney beans.

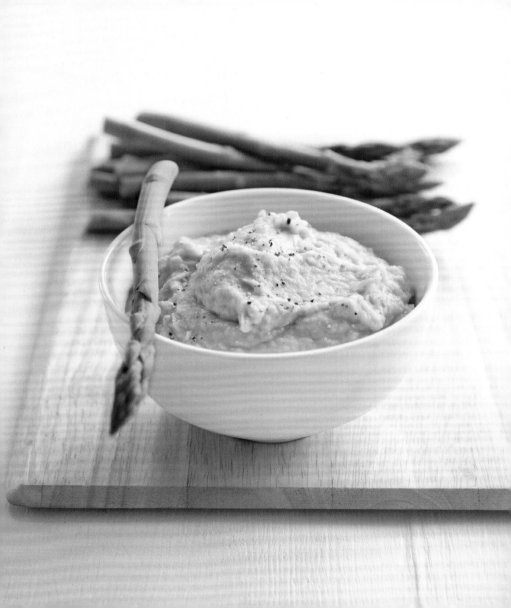

beet & orange hummus

Serves **4**

2 (15 oz) cans **chickpeas (garbanzo beans)**, drained
3 **garlic cloves,** peeled
1½ tablespoons **tahini**
1 **beet**
1 **orange**, coarsely peeled
2–3 tablespoons **olive oil**
salt and **black pepper**
oatcakes or **crispbreads**,
 to serve

Put the chickpeas and garlic cloves into a food processor or blender and process until broken down. Add the tahini and process for another 5–10 seconds.

Juice the beet with the orange. Pour the juice into the food processor or blender and process again, gradually adding the olive oil until you have the consistency you prefer. Season to taste and serve with oatcakes or crispbreads.

For cilantro hummus, follow the recipe above, omitting the beet and adding a small handful of cilantro leaves to the food processor or blender with the chickpeas and garlic.

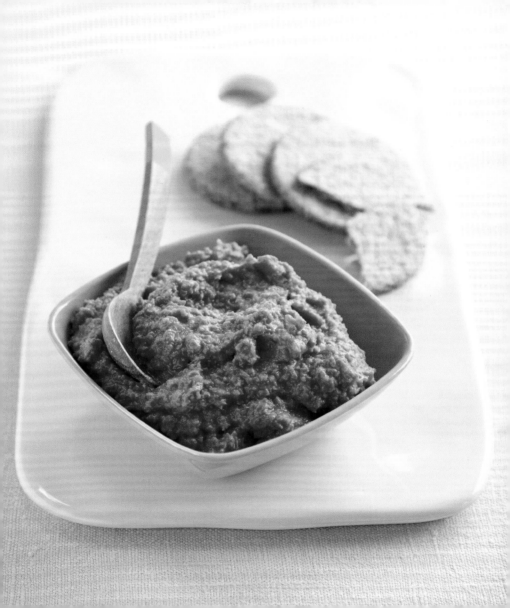

blue cheese & celery dip

Serves **2**

3 **celery sticks**
5 oz **blue cheese**
vegetable crudités, to serve

Juice the celery.

Transfer the celery juice to a food processor or blender, add the cheese, and process until smooth. Serve with vegetable crudités.

For cream cheese & red pepper dip, juice 1 cored and seeded red bell pepper. Pour the juice into a small bowl, add 1 cup cream cheese (or more depending on your preferred thickness of dip), and stir to combine.

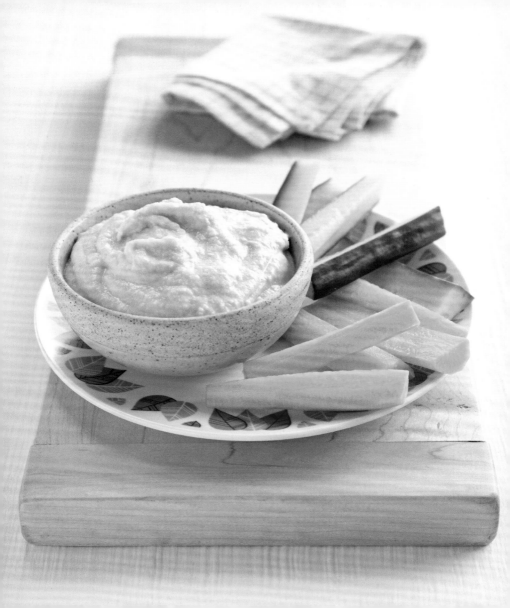

arugula & macadamia nut dip

Serves **2**

½ **celery stick**
1 ¼ cups **spinach**
¾ cup **arugula**
⅓ cup **macadamia nuts**
½ **garlic clove**, peeled
1 tablespoon grated
  Parmesan
1–2 tablespoons **olive oil**
salt and **black pepper**
toasted **pita bread**, to serve

Juice the celery with the spinach.

Transfer the juice to a food processor or blender, add the arugula, macadamia nuts, garlic, and Parmesan and process until smooth, gradually adding the olive oil until you have the consistency you prefer. Season to taste and serve with toasted pita bread.

For watercress & walnut dip, follow the recipe above, replacing the arugula with 8 sprigs of watercress and the macadamia nuts with ½ cup walnuts.

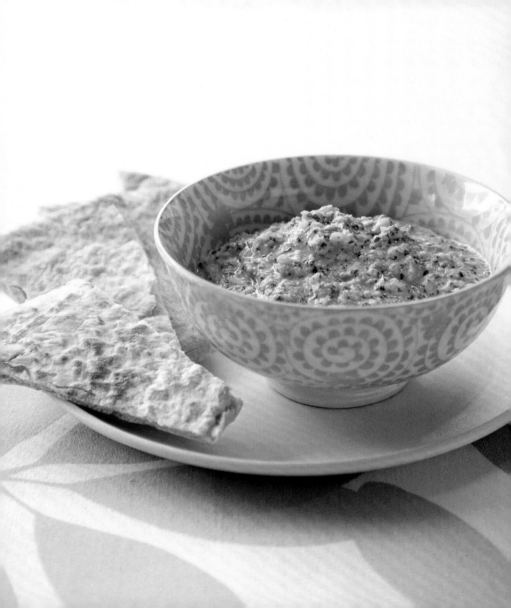

tomato salsa

Serves **4**

4 large **tomatoes**
½ **lime**, coarsely peeled
½ **red bell pepper**, cored and
  seeded
1 **green chile**, finely chopped
½ medium **red onion**, diced
½ cup chopped **cilantro**
  leaves
salt and **black pepper**
tortilla chips, to serve

Score a cross into the bottom of each tomato with a sharp knife and put into a large bowl. Pour over enough boiling water to cover and let stand for 20 seconds. Transfer the tomatoes to a bowl of iced water, using a slotted spoon, and let cool slightly. When cool, peel off the skins. Cut the tomatoes in half, remove and discard the seeds, and chop the tomato flesh.

Juice the lime with the red bell pepper. Transfer the juice to a bowl.

Add the chopped tomatoes to the juice along with the chile, red onion, and cilantro. Stir to combine and season to taste. Serve with tortilla chips.

For avocado & tomato salsa, follow the recipe above, replacing 2 of the tomatoes with 1 large avocado. Peel, pit, and dice the avocado and stir into the salsa with the chile, onion, and cilantro.

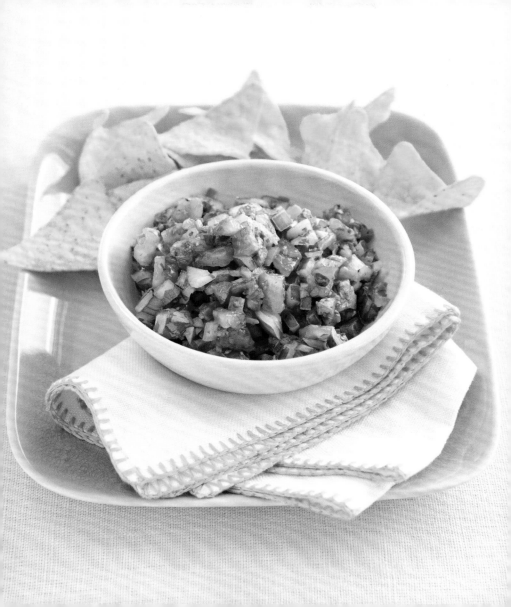

asparagus, feta & white bean dip

Serves **2**

8 **asparagus spears**
1 (15 oz) can **cannellini
(white kidney) beans**,
  drained
1 **garlic clove**, peeled
⅓ cup **feta cheese**
1 tablespoon **olive oil**
black pepper
cooked jumbo shrimp,
  to serve

Juice the asparagus.

Transfer the juice to a food processor or blender, add the beans, garlic, feta, and olive oil, and process until smooth. Season to taste and serve with jumbo shrimp for dipping.

For tomato & lima bean dip, juice 2 large tomatoes. Transfer the juice to a food processor or blender, add 1 (15 oz) drained can lima beans, ¼ cup parsley, and 1 peeled garlic clove, and process until smooth, gradually adding olive oil until you have the consistency you prefer. Season to taste and serve.

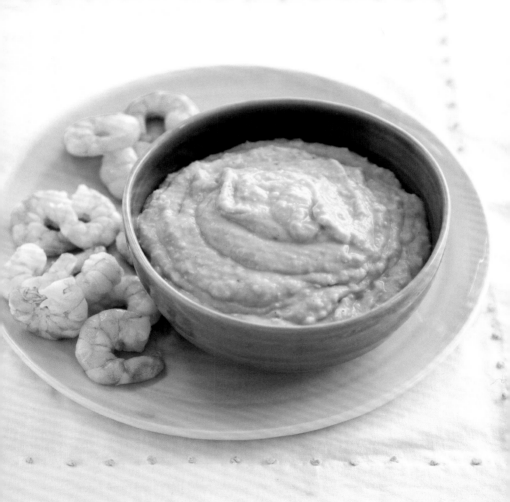

french onion dip

Serves **2**

1 ½ teaspoons **olive oil**

4 **onions**, peeled and finely chopped

1 **garlic clove**, crushed

1 ½ teaspoons **Worcestershire sauce**

leaves from 2 **thyme sprigs**

1 cup **Greek yogurt**

¾ inch piece fresh **horseradish root**, peeled

salt and **black pepper**

Heat the oil in a skillet. Add the onions and cook over low heat for 18–20 minutes, stirring from time to time, until they start to caramelize and turn golden. Stir in the crushed garlic and cook for another 2 minutes, then stir in the Worcestershire sauce and thyme and remove from the heat. Let cool.

Transfer the onion mixture to a serving bowl and stir in the yogurt.

Juice the horseradish and add the juice to the onion dip. Season to taste and serve.

For celery & onion dip, follow the recipe above, replacing 2 of the onions with 3 finely sliced celery sticks and omitting the thyme.

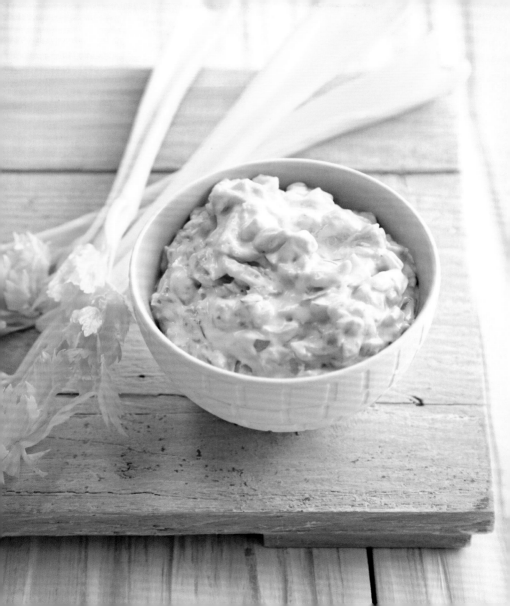

digestive dip

Serves **2**

1 **lime**
2 **papaya**, peeled and seeded
½ cup **plain yogurt**
fresh fruit, to serve

Grate the zest of the lime and reserve. Juice the lime.

Transfer the juice to a food processor or blender, add the papaya and yogurt, and process until smooth. Stir in the reserved grated lime zest. Serve with fresh fruit for dipping.

For lime & apple dip, prepare the lime as above. Pour the lime juice into a bowl and add 1 cup plain yogurt with 2 grated apples. Mix to combine. Stir in the grated lime zest and a large pinch of cinnamon. Serve with fresh fruit for dipping.

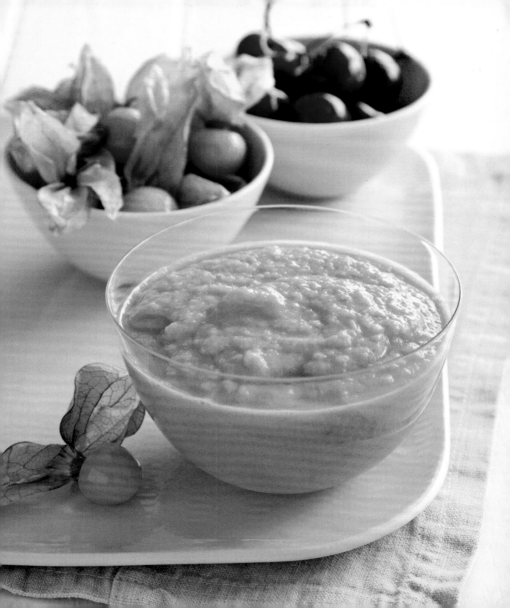

satay dip

Serves **2**

1 **lime**, coarsely peeled
¾ inch piece fresh **ginger root**, peeled
1 **garlic clove**, peeled
3 tablespoons **smooth peanut butter**
3–4 tablespoons **coconut milk**
½ teaspoon **soy sauce**
1 tablespoon chopped **cilantro leaves**
chicken kebabs, to serve

Juice the lime with the ginger.

Transfer the juice to a food processor or blender, add the garlic, peanut butter, coconut milk, and soy sauce, and process until combined. Stir in the chopped cilantro. Serve with chicken kebabs.

For hot & crunchy satay dip, follow the recipe above, adding 1 red chile to the blender with the other ingredients and stirring 1 tablespoon chopped hazelnuts into the dip with the chopped cilantro.

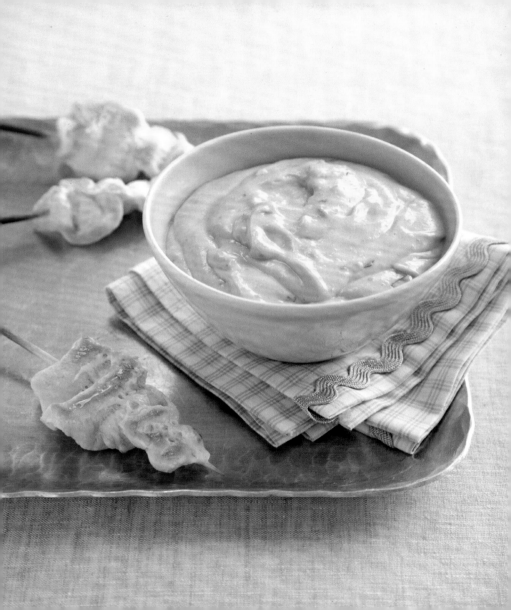

carrot & cashew dip

Serves **4**

2 **oranges**, coarsely peeled
2 **carrots**, peeled and
  thinly sliced
1 tablespoon **cashew nuts**
8 **dried apricots**, diced
1 teaspoon **cumin seeds**

Juice the oranges.

Put the carrots into a saucepan with half the orange juice, add water to cover, if necessary, bring to a boil, and simmer for 10 minutes. Add the cashews and apricots, cover, and cook for another 5–7 minutes, until the carrots are just tender.

Meanwhile, put the cumin seeds into a skillet and toast over high heat for 1–2 minutes. Grind the toasted seeds briefly in a mortar and pestle.

Put the carrot mixture into a food processor or blender, add the remaining orange juice, and process until smooth. Transfer to a bowl and chill for at least an hour and serve sprinkled with the ground cumin seeds.

For lemony cashew dip, soak ¼ cup cashew nuts in water for 2 hours to soften. Juice 1 coarsely peeled lemon. Transfer the lemon juice to a food processor or blender, add the drained cashew nuts, 1 tablespoon tahini, and 1 peeled garlic clove, and process until smooth, gradually adding olive oil until you have the consistency you prefer.

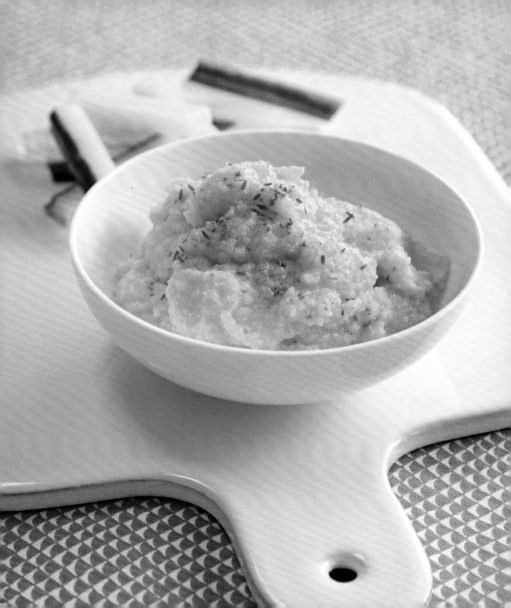

chocolate & orange dip

Serves **2**

1 **orange**
2 tablespoons **cocoa nibs**
1 large **avocado**
½ teaspoon **honey**
apple and **pear** slices,
   to serve

Grate the zest of the orange and reserve. Coarsely peel and then juice the orange.

Grind the cocoa nibs to a powder. Peel and pit the avocado.

Transfer the orange juice, cocoa powder, avocado, and honey to a blender or food processor and process until smooth. Stir in the grated orange zest. Serve with slices of apple and pear.

For orange & mango dip, prepare the orange as above. Transfer the orange juice, 1 large peeled and pitted avocado, 1 large peeled and pitted mango, and a ¾ inch piece preserved ginger to a food processor or blender and process until smooth.

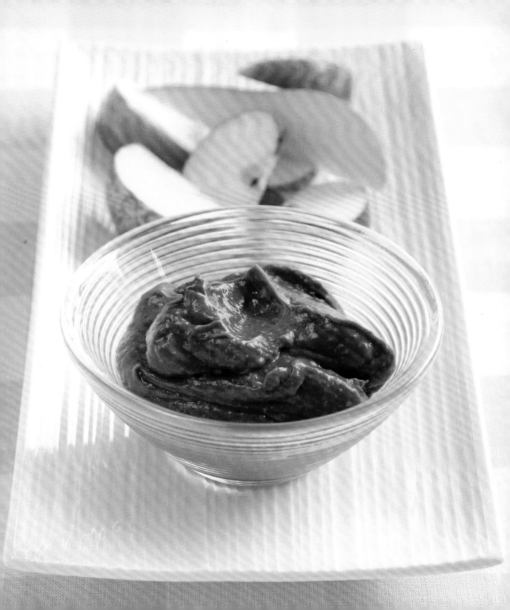

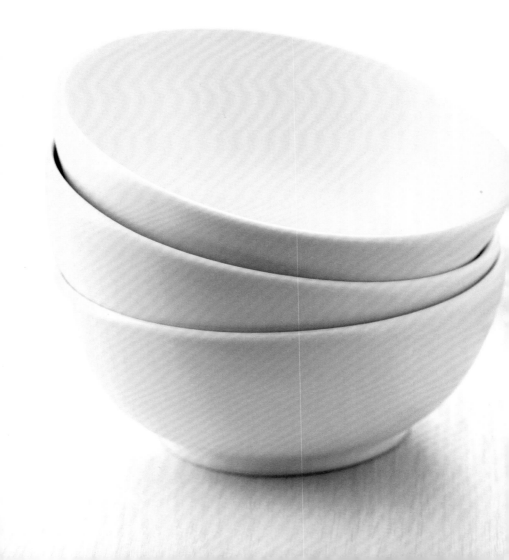

juicy soups

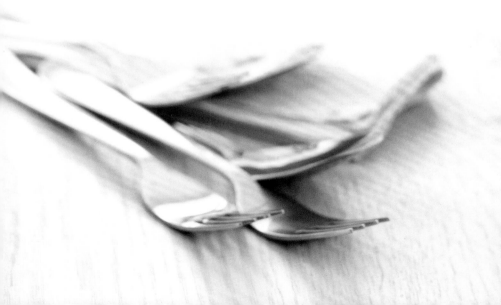

green gazpacho

Serves **4**

1 **lime**, coarsely peeled

1 large **tomato**

1 **cucumber**, coarsely chopped

1 **yellow bell pepper**, cored and seeded

2 **garlic cloves**, chopped

1 **avocado**, peeled and pitted

6 **scallions**, trimmed and coarsely chopped

⅓ cup **mint**

½ cup **plain yogurt**

8 **ice cubes**

2 tablespoons **extra virgin olive oil**

chopped **chives**, to garnish

Juice the lime with the tomato.

Transfer the juice to a food processor or blender, add the cucumber, yellow bell pepper, garlic, avocado, scallions, mint, and yogurt, and process until nearly smooth. Chill until cold.

Ladle the soup into bowls, add a couple of ice cubes to each bowl, drizzle with extra virgin olive oil, and garnish with the chopped chives.

For tomato gazpacho, juice the lime and tomato as above. Transfer the juice to a food processor or blender, add 1 coarsely chopped cucumber, 1 cored and seeded red bell pepper, 2 chopped garlic cloves, 6 trimmed and coarsely chopped scallions, 4 coarsely chopped tomatoes, ¼ cup basil, and 2 tablespoons olive oil, and process until nearly smooth. Chill until cold. Serve garnished with 1 peeled, pitted, and diced avocado.

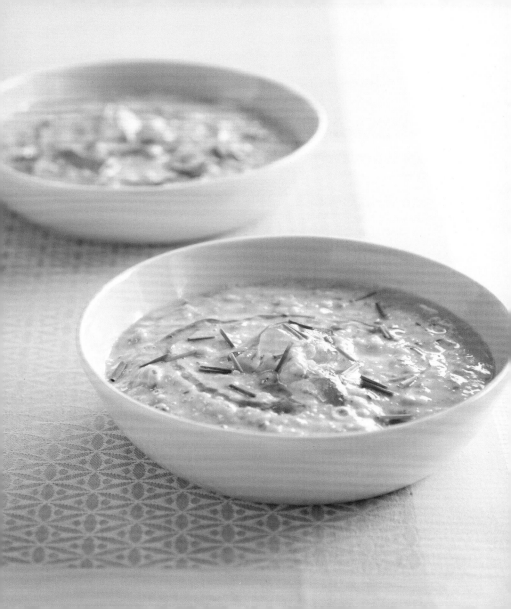

carrot, lentil & orange soup

Serves **4**

3 **oranges**, coarsely peeled
1 teaspoon **cumin seeds**
1 teaspoon **mustard seeds**
1 teaspoon **coriander seeds**
1 **onion**, peeled and diced
4 **carrots**, peeled and diced
⅓ cup **red lentils**
2½ cups **vegetable broth**
2 tablespoons **plain yogurt**
cilantro sprigs, to garnish

Juice the oranges.

Dry-fry the spices in a saucepan over medium heat for 1–2 minutes. Add the onion, carrots, red lentils, orange juice, and vegetable broth, bring to a boil, and simmer for 25–30 minutes, until the carrots are tender and the lentils are soft.

Transfer the soup, in batches, to a food processor or blender and process until smooth, transferring each successive batch to a clean saucepan. Heat through gently.

Ladle the soup into bowls, top with a swirl of yogurt, and garnish with cilantro sprigs.

For carrot & cilantro soup, make as above but increase the carrots to 5 large carrots and omit the lentils. Stir ¼ cup cilantro leaves into the soup before blending. Serve with plain yogurt and a sprinkling of paprika.

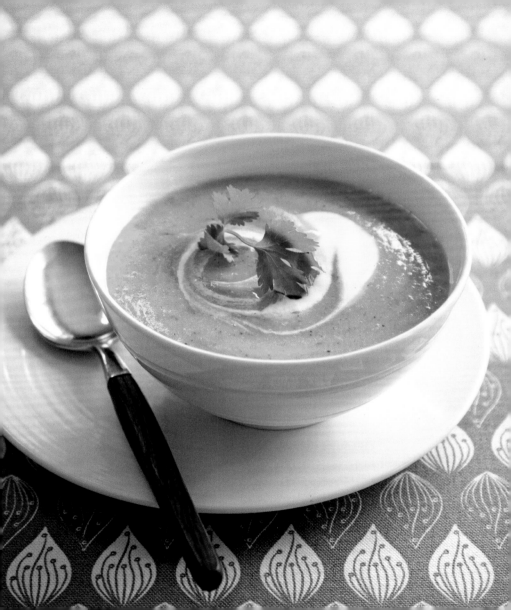

roasted pepper & tomato soup

Serves **2**

4 **red bell peppers**,
   cored and seeded
4 **tomatoes**, halved
1 teaspoon **olive oil**
1 **onion**, chopped
1 **carrot**, chopped
2½ cups **vegetable broth**
2 tablespoons **crème fraîche**
   or **Greek yogurt**
handful of **basil leaves**, torn
black pepper

Put the bell peppers, skin side up, and the tomatoes, skin side down, onto a baking sheet under a hot broiler and cook for 8–10 minutes, until the skins of the bell peppers are blackened. Cover the bell peppers with damp paper towels, let cool, then remove the paper along with the skins and slice the flesh. Let the tomatoes cool, then remove the skins.

Heat the oil in a large saucepan, add the onion and carrot, and sauté for 5 minutes. Add the broth and the skinned roasted peppers and tomatoes, bring to a boil, and simmer for 20 minutes, until the carrot is tender.

Transfer the soup, in batches, to a food processor or blender and process until smooth, transferring each successive batch to a clean saucepan. Heat through gently. Stir through the crème fraîche or yogurt and basil and season well with black pepper.

Ladle the soup into bowls and serve.

For roasted zucchini & pea soup, replace the red bell peppers with 4 medium zucchini, sliced lengthwise and roasted as above. Add 1⅓ cups frozen peas with the broth and bring to a boil. Season to taste and garnish with torn basil and mint leaves.

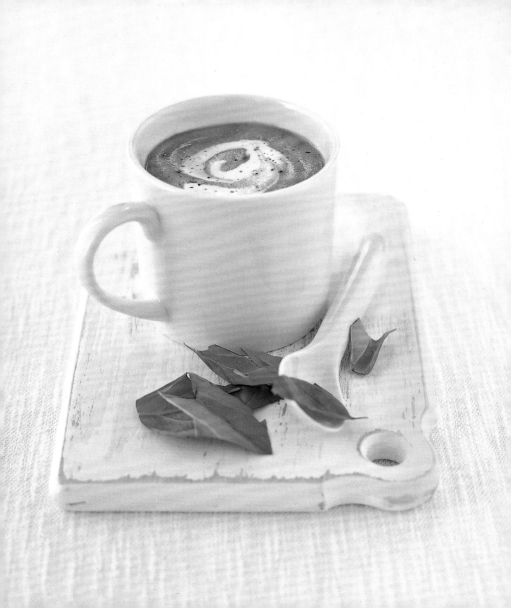

pistou soup

Serves **4**

1 tablespoon **olive oil**
1 **onion**, peeled and diced
1 **leek**, trimmed and sliced
1 **celery stick**, diced
2 **carrots**, peeled and diced
1 small **fennel bulb**, trimmed
and diced
½ **celeriac (celery root)**,
peeled and diced
1 cup **frozen peas**
1 (15 oz) can **navy beans**,
drained
1¼ cups **spinach**
¼ cup **pesto**
salt and **black pepper**
basil leaves, to garnish

Heat the oil in a saucepan. Add the onion, leek, celery, carrots, fennel, and celeriac and cook gently over low heat for 8–10 minutes, until starting to soften but not browned. Pour in 4 cups of boiling water and season with salt and black pepper. Bring to a boil and simmer for 10–15 minutes, adding the peas and beans for the last minute of cooking.

Meanwhile, juice the spinach. Pour the juice into a small bowl, add the pesto, and stir to combine.

Ladle the soup into bowls, stir a spoonful of the pesto into each bowl of soup, and garnish with a few basil leaves.

For winter vegetable soup, heat 1 tablespoon olive oil in a saucepan. Add 1 peeled and chopped onion, 2 trimmed and sliced leeks, 2 peeled and diced carrots, 2 cups peeled and diced rutabaga, and 2 peeled and diced parsnips and cook gently over low heat for 8–10 minutes, until starting to soften but not browned. Pour in 4 cups of vegetable broth, bring to a boil, and simmer for 12–15 minutes. Season to taste. Juice ½ bunch of watercress. Pour the juice into a small bowl, add ¼ cup red pesto, and stir to combine. Ladle the soup into bowls and stir a spoonful of the pesto into each bowl of soup.

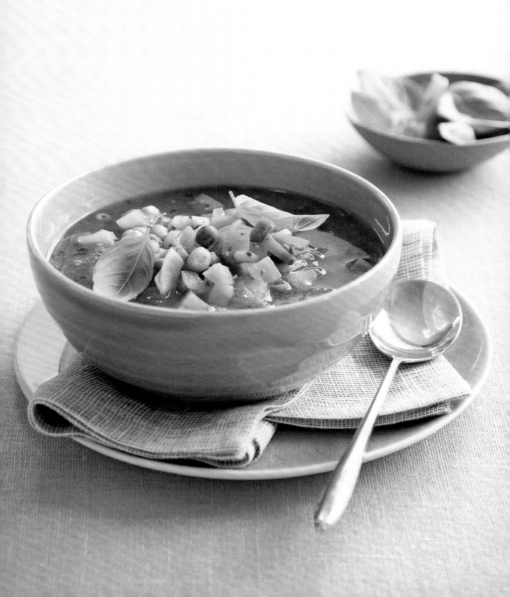

salmon & horseradish soup

Serves **4**

1 tablespoon **olive oil**
1 **leek**, trimmed and sliced
4 **Yukon gold** or **white round potatoes**, peeled and chopped
4 cups **fish broth**
9 oz **salmon fillet**, cut into bite-size chunks
2 tablespoons **plain yogurt**
¾ inch piece fresh **horseradish root**
salt and **black pepper**
chopped chives, to garnish

Heat the oil in a large saucepan. Add the leek and sauté for 3–4 minutes. Then stir in the potatoes, pour in the broth, bring to a boil, and simmer for 12–15 minutes, until the potatoes are tender. Stir in half the salmon chunks and cook for another 2 minutes.

Add the yogurt and stir through. Transfer the soup, in batches, to a food processor or blender and process until smooth, transferring each successive batch to a clean saucepan.

Juice the horseradish. Pour the juice into the soup, add the remaining salmon chunks, and heat through gently. Season with salt and black pepper.

Ladle the soup into bowls and garnish with some chopped chives.

For chunky salmon soup, heat 1 tablespoon olive oil in a saucepan. Add 2 trimmed and sliced leeks and sauté for 2 minutes, then add 1 large, peeled and diced potato, ⅓ cup red lentils and 3 cups skim milk, bring to a boil, and simmer for 25–30 minutes. Stir in 7 oz salmon fillet, cut into chunks, and cook for 2–3 minutes more. Juice a ¾ inch piece of fresh ginger root and stir the juice into the soup. Season to taste and serve sprinkled with chopped parsley.

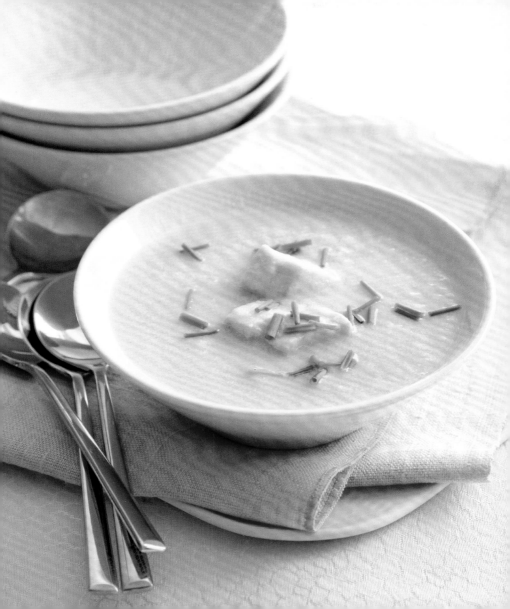

bean soup with guacamole

1 teaspoon **olive oil**
1 **onion**, chopped
1 **garlic clove**, crushed
1 **red chile**, seeded and
  chopped
2 cups rinsed and drained
  canned **mixed beans**,
  such as kidney beans, pinto
  beans, and chickpeas
1 cup canned **diced tomatoes**
1¼ cups **vegetable broth**
salt and **black pepper**
tortilla chips, to serve

Guacamole
1 **avocado**, skinned and pitted
2 **scallions**, finely sliced
2 **tomatoes**, chopped
1 tablespoon chopped
  cilantro leaves
juice of ½ **lime**

Make the guacamole. Coarsely chop the avocado flesh and mash it together with the scallions, tomatoes, cilantro, and lime juice. Set aside.

Heat the oil in a medium saucepan. Add the onion, garlic, and chile and sauté for 2–3 minutes or until softened. Add the beans, tomatoes, and broth, bring to a boil, and simmer for 10 minutes.

Transfer three-quarters of the soup to a food processor or blender and process until almost smooth. Add to the reserved soup and stir to combine. Season to taste with salt and black pepper and heat through gently.

Serve the soup with the guacamole and tortilla chips.

For smoked bacon & bean soup with guacamole, add 2 oz chopped smoked bacon to the saucepan with the onion, garlic, and chile and cook for 2–3 minutes. Continue as above. Garnish with a spoonful of sour cream and serve with the guacamole.

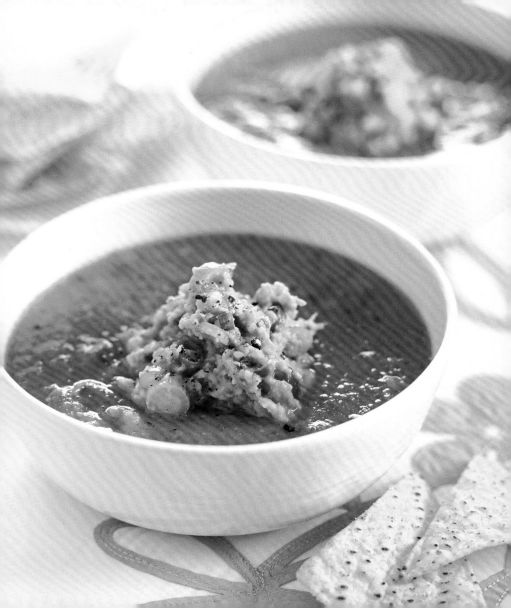

chilled avocado & broccoli soup

Serves **4**

1 **lime**, coarsely peeled
2 cups **broccoli florets**
1 **cucumber**, coarsely
   chopped
2 **garlic cloves**
2 large **avocados**, peeled
   and pitted
4 **tomatoes**
6–8 **basil leaves**
salt and **black pepper**

Juice the lime with the broccoli.

Put the cucumber, garlic, avocado, and half of the tomatoes and basil into a food processor or blender. Pour in the juice and process until smooth, adding a little water to loosen the mixture, if necessary. Season to taste and chill for at least 30 minutes before serving.

Finely chop the remaining tomatoes and basil leaves. Ladle the soup into bowls and serve sprinkled with the chopped tomatoes and basil.

For chilled cucumber soup, juice ½ lemon with 1 celery stick. Transfer the juice to a food processor or blender, add 3 cucumbers, 1 red chile (optional), a small handful of mint leaves, and 3 ice cubes, and process until smooth. Season to taste and serve with a drizzle of avocado oil.

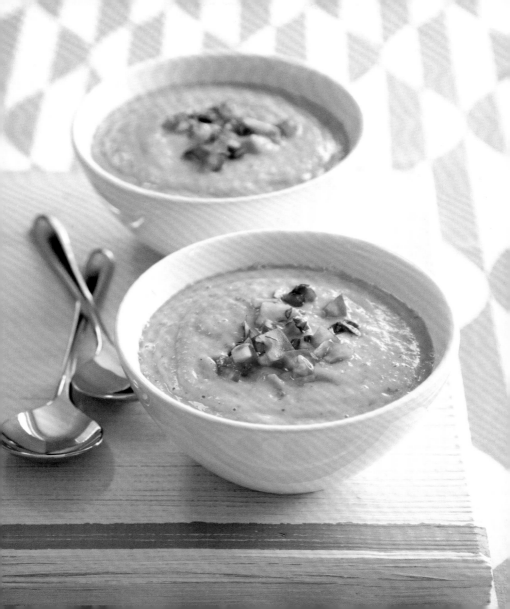

chicken & sweet potato soup

Serves **2**

2 teaspoons **olive oil**
1 **small onion**, chopped
1 **garlic clove**, crushed
1 **red chile**, seeded and
  chopped
1 large **sweet potato**, peeled
  and cubed
1 large boneless, skinless
  chicken breast, chopped
1 (15 oz) can **coconut milk**
2½ cups **chicken broth**
1 tablespoon chopped
  cilantro leaves
salt

Heat the oil in a nonstick skillet. Add the onion, garlic, and chile, and sauté for 3 minutes, until softened. Add the sweet potato and chicken and continue to cook for 2–3 minutes, until the chicken is browned all over. Add the coconut milk and broth to the pan, bring to a boil, cover, and simmer for 15 minutes, until the potato is tender.

Transfer the soup, in batches, to a food processor or blender and process until smooth, transferring each successive batch to a clean saucepan. Heat through gently. Season to taste with salt, stir through the chopped cilantro, and serve.

For spiced butternut squash soup, cook the onion, garlic, and chile as above, but omit the chicken and replace the sweet potato with 1 medium peeled and chopped butternut squash. Add the coconut milk and 1¼ cups vegetable broth instead of the chicken broth. Bring to a boil and finish as above.

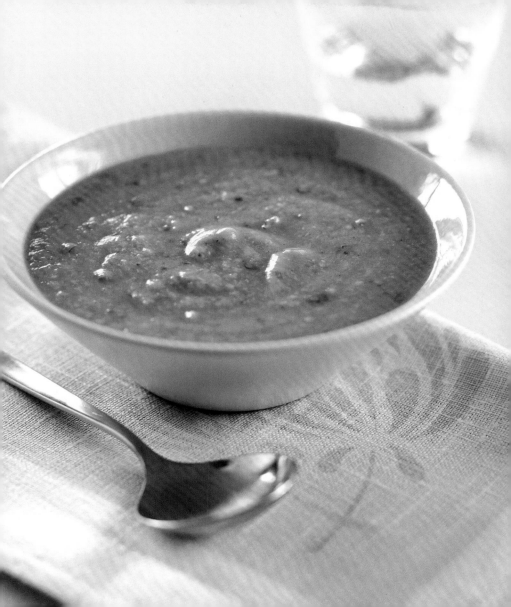

beet & horseradish soup

Serves **4**

1 tablespoon **sunflower oil**
1 **red onion**, peeled and
  chopped
1 **celery stick**, chopped
1 tablespoon chopped **thyme**
6 **beets**, peeled and cut into
  small chunks
1 tablespoon **red wine
  vinegar**
3¾ cups hot **vegetable broth**
2 tablespoons **creamed
  horseradish sauce**, plus
  2 teaspoons
salt and **black pepper**
crusty bread, to serve

To garnish
3 tablespoons **sour cream**
  or **crème fraîche**
chopped chives

Heat the oil in a large saucepan, add the onion, celery, and thyme, and cook gently for 3–4 minutes. Add the beets and vinegar and cook for 2 minutes.

Pour in the broth, cover, and simmer for about 25 minutes, until the beets are tender. Season to taste with salt and black pepper and stir in 2 tablespoons of horseradish sauce.

Transfer the soup, in batches, to a food processor or blender and process until smooth, transferring each successive batch to a clean saucepan. Heat through gently.

Ladle the soup into bowls. Mix the sour cream or crème fraîche with the remaining horseradish sauce and spoon on top of the soup. Garnish with chopped chives and serve with crusty bread, if desired.

For beet & caraway soup, heat 1 tablespoon sunflower oil in a large saucepan, add 1 chopped onion and 1 crushed garlic clove, and cook gently for 3–4 minutes, until softened. Stir in 1 teaspoon caraway seeds, 6 beets, peeled and diced, 1 medium potato, peeled and diced, 1 tablespoon apple cider vinegar, and 3¾ cups vegetable broth. Cover and simmer for 30 minutes, until the beets and potato are tender. Season to taste with salt and black pepper, then transfer the soup, in batches, to a food processor or blender and process until smooth, transferring each successive batch to a clean saucepan. Heat through gently. Serve topped with a spoonful of Greek yogurt and a sprinkling of caraway seeds.

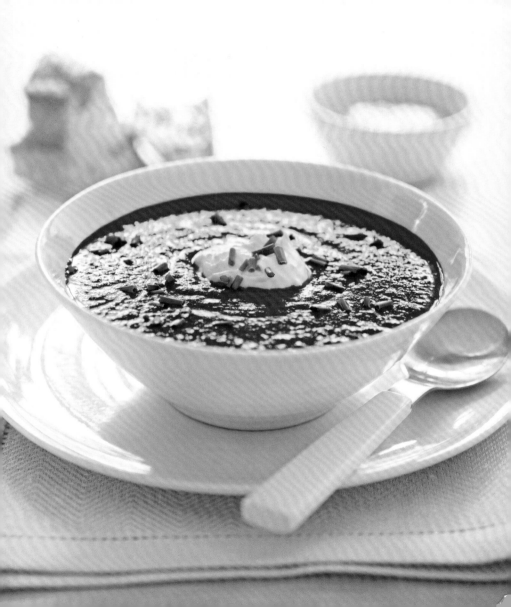

broccoli & cheddar soup

Serves **2**

1½ bunches of **broccoli**
1 tablespoon **olive oil**
1 **onion**, chopped
1 **large potato**, peeled and
  quartered
6⅓ cups **vegetable broth**
½ cup **crème fraîche** or
  sour cream
1 tablespoon **lemon juice**
1 teaspoon **Worcestershire
  sauce**
a few drops of **Tabasco
  sauce**
1 cup shredded **sharp
  cheddar cheese**
salt and **black pepper**
watercress, to garnish

Remove all the tough stems and leaves from the broccoli. Cut off the remaining stems, peel them, and cut into 1 inch pieces. Break the florets into small pieces and set them aside.

Heat the olive oil in a large saucepan. Add the onion and broccoli stems and cook, covered, for 5 minutes over medium heat, stirring frequently.

Add the broccoli florets, potato, and vegetable broth to the pan. Bring the mixture to a boil, season, and cook, partly covered, for 25 minutes, or until all the vegetables are soft.

Transfer the soup, in batches, to a food processor or blender and process until smooth, transferring each successive batch to a clean saucepan. Chill until required.

When ready to serve, add the crème fraîche or sour cream, lemon juice, Worcestershire sauce, and a few drops of Tabasco to the pan. Heat the soup gently and simmer for 3–5 minutes, but do not let the soup boil. Just before serving, stir in the shredded cheddar. Serve the soup, garnished with watercress.

For creamy cauliflower & cheddar soup, cut 1 large cauliflower into small florets. Sauté in 1 tablespoon olive oil with 1 chopped onion as above. Add 2½ cups vegetable broth, season, and simmer for 10 minutes. Puree, in batches, and return to the pan. Chill until required. Stir in 2 cups milk, 2 teaspoons Dijon mustard, and a little grated nutmeg. Reheat and stir in ¾ cup shredded cheddar cheese.

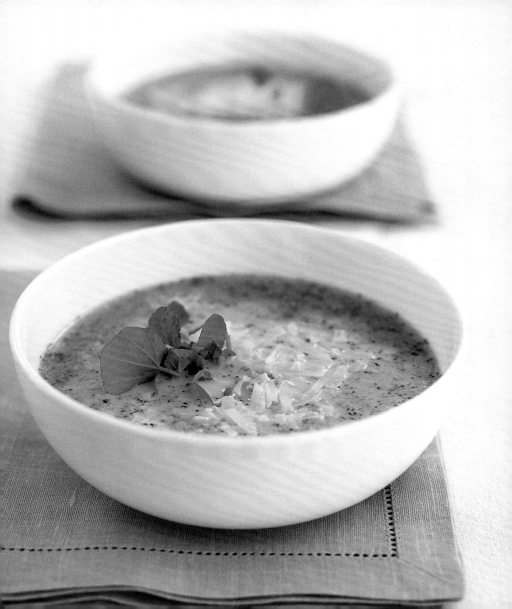

curried parsnip soup

Serves **4**

1 tablespoon **olive oil**
1 **onion**, chopped
2 **garlic cloves**, crushed
1 inch piece of fresh **ginger root**, peeled and chopped
1 tablespoon **medium curry powder**
1 teaspoon **cumin seeds**
6 **parsnips**, peeled and chopped
4 cups **vegetable broth**
salt and **black pepper**

To serve
plain yogurt
2 tablespoons chopped **cilantro leaves**
naan or other **flatbread**, warmed

Heat the olive oil in a large saucepan, add the onion, garlic, and ginger, and cook over medium heat for 4–5 minutes, until softened.

Stir in the curry powder and cumin seeds and cook, stirring, for 2 minutes, then stir in the parsnips, making sure that they are well coated in the spice mixture. Pour in the broth and bring to a boil, then cover and simmer for 20–25 minutes, until the parsnips are tender. Season to taste with salt and black pepper.

Transfer the soup, in batches, to a food processor or blender and process until smooth, transferring each successive batch to a clean saucepan. Heat through gently. Serve in cups with dollops of yogurt, garnished with the cilantro and with warm naan or other flatbread.

For caramelized parsnip & honey soup, heat 1 tablespoon olive oil in a flameproof roasting pan on the stove, add the peeled and chopped parsnips and 2 thyme sprigs, and turn to coat in the oil. Roast in a preheated oven, at 400°F, for 30–35 minutes, stirring once, until golden brown. Stir in 2 tablespoons honey and roast for another 10 minutes, until the parsnips have caramelized. Transfer to a saucepan, stir in 4 cups vegetable broth, and bring to a boil on the stove, then simmer for 10 minutes. Transfer to a food processor or blender, in batches, and process until smooth. Return to the pan, season to taste, and stir in 1 ¼ cups boiling water, then bring back to a boil. Serve in bowls with crusty bread.

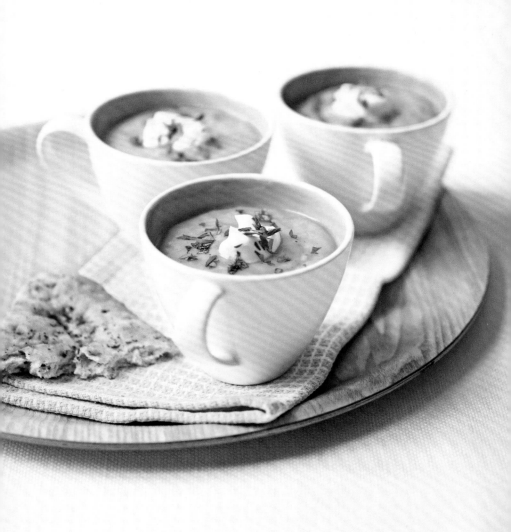

potato & smoked garlic soup

Serves **4**

1 tablespoon **olive oil**

1 **large onion**, sliced

2 smoked **garlic cloves**, crushed

6 **Yukon gold** or **white round potatoes**, peeled and cut into small cubes

4 cups **vegetable broth**

½ teaspoon **smoked sea salt**

½ cup **milk**

¼ cup **fresh herbs**, such as parsley, thyme, and chives, plus extra snipped chives, to garnish

black pepper

Greek yogurt, to serve

Heat the olive oil in a large saucepan, add the onion and smoked garlic, and cook over medium heat for 3–4 minutes, until softened. Stir in the potatoes, cover, and cook for 5 minutes.

Add the broth and season with the smoked sea salt and black pepper. Bring to a boil, then reduce the heat, cover, and simmer for 30 minutes, until the potatoes are tender.

Transfer the soup, in batches, to a food processor or blender and process until smooth, transferring each successive batch to a clean saucepan. Stir in the milk and herbs and reheat gently.

Ladle the soup into bowls, add a spoonful of Greek yogurt, and garnish with chives and black pepper.

For smoked sweet potato soup, cook the onion and garlic as above, then add 1 tablespoon smoked paprika and cook, stirring, for 1 minute. Stir in 3 Yukon gold or white round potatoes and 3 sweet potatoes, both peeled and cut into small cubes, and cook for 5 minutes. Add the broth as above and bring to a boil, then cover and simmer for 30 minutes, until the potato is tender. Blend as above until smooth, then serve with a spoonful of Greek yogurt, garnished with a sprinkling of smoked paprika and freshly snipped chives.

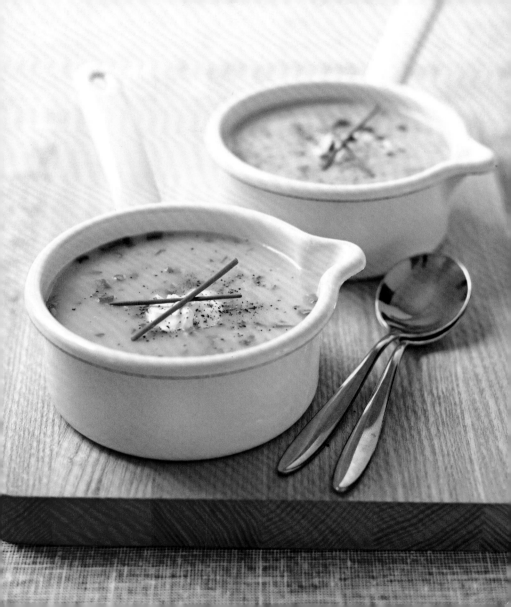

tomato & chorizo soup

Serves **2**

4 **red bell peppers**, cored
  and seeded
2 tablespoons **olive oil**
1 **large onion**, chopped
2 **garlic cloves**, crushed
5 oz **chorizo sausage**, sliced
1 teaspoon ground **cumin**
1 teaspoon **smoked paprika**
4 **tomatoes**, halved and
  seeded
2½ cups **chicken** or
  vegetable broth
handful of **parsley**, chopped
salt and **black pepper**

Put the red bell peppers onto a baking sheet and drizzle with half the olive oil. Place in a preheated oven, at 400°F, for 10–15 minutes, turning after 5 minutes.

Heat the remaining olive oil in a large saucepan, while the bell peppers are roasting, add the onion, garlic, and chorizo, and sauté for 3–4 minutes, until the onion is softened and the chorizo is beginning to brown. Stir in the spices and cook for another minute.

Add the tomatoes and broth to the saucepan and season well. Bring to a boil and simmer for 5 minutes.

Remove the red bell peppers from the oven. Skin and coarsely chop them, then add to the soup and simmer for another 15 minutes. Remove from the heat and let cool for 5 minutes.

Transfer the soup, in batches, to a food processor or blender and coarsely blend, transferring each successive batch to a clean saucepan. Heat through gently, then stir in the parsley and serve.

For tomato soup with creamy basil, omit the red bell peppers and sauté the onion and garlic as above, replacing the chorizo and spices with 1 chopped carrot and 1 chopped celery stick. Add the tomatoes and vegetable broth, bring to a boil, and simmer for 25 minutes. Transfer the soup, in batches, to a food processor or blender and process until smooth, transferring each successive batch to a clean saucepan. Heat through gently and stir in 2 tablespoons mascarpone cheese and 1 tablespoon pesto. Season and serve.

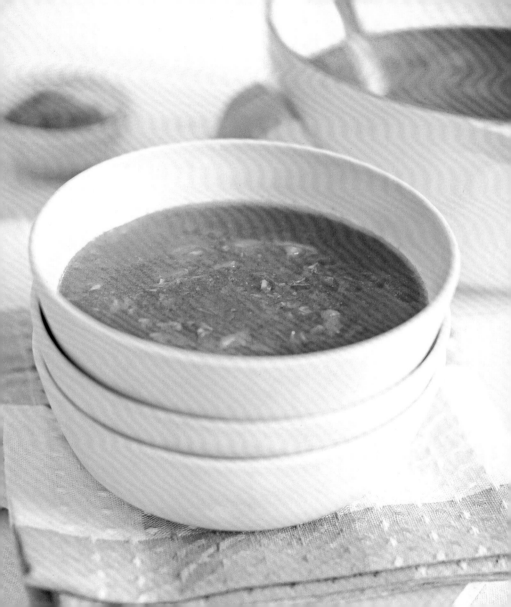

bacon & white bean soup

Serves **4**

1 teaspoon **olive oil**

2 lean **smoked bacon slices**, chopped

2 **garlic cloves**, crushed

1 **onion**, chopped

a few **thyme** or **lemon thyme sprigs**

2 (15 oz) cans **cannellini (white kidney) beans**, drained and rinsed

3¾ cups **vegetable broth**

2 tablespoons chopped **parsley**

black pepper

Heat the oil in a large saucepan, add the bacon, garlic, and onion, and sauté for 3–4 minutes, until the bacon is beginning to brown and the onion to soften.

Add the thyme and cook for another 1 minute. Add the beans and broth to the pan and bring to a boil, then reduce the heat and simmer for 10 minutes.

Transfer the soup, in batches, to a food processor or blender with the parsley and black pepper and process until smooth, transferring each successive batch to a clean saucepan. Heat through gently and serve.

For herb & white bean crostini, to serve as an accompaniment, lightly mash 1 (15 oz) can drained cannellini (white kidney) beans and then combine with 2 tablespoons each of finely chopped basil and parsley, 1 crushed garlic clove, a pinch of dried red pepper flakes, and 3 chopped cherry tomatoes. Toast 8 thin slices of baguette and top with the herb bean mixture.

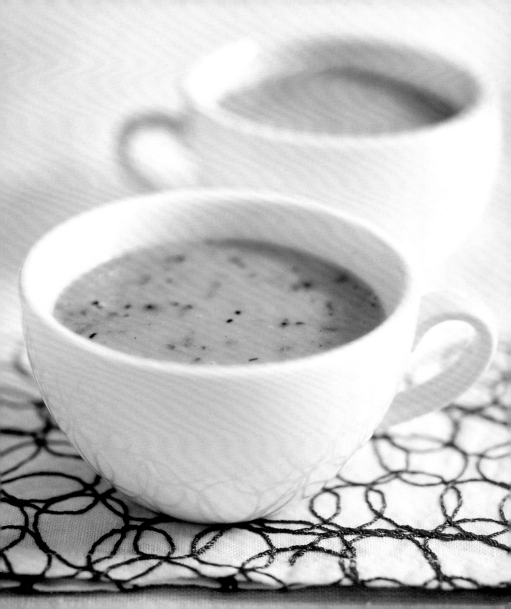

green detox soup

Serves **4**

1 tablespoon **coconut oil**

1 large **onion**, peeled and chopped

1 **leek**, trimmed and sliced

2 **garlic cloves**, crushed

¾ inch piece fresh **ginger root**, peeled and diced

1 teaspoon **cumin seeds**

½ teaspoon ground **turmeric**

2 cups coarsely chopped **savoy cabbage**

2 cups **broccoli florets**

1 **parsnip**, peeled and chopped

3¾ cups **vegetable broth**

1 **lemon**

2 cups **spinach**

salt and **black pepper**

2 tablespoons **plain yogurt**

chopped **cilantro leaves**

Heat the oil in a large saucepan, add the onion and leek, and sauté for 4–5 minutes. Stir in the garlic, ginger, and spices and cook for 1–2 minutes, then stir in the cabbage, broccoli, and parsnip and cook for another 1 minute. Add the broth, bring to a boil, and simmer for 12–15 minutes, until the parsnip is soft.

Transfer the soup, in batches, to a food processor or blender and process until smooth, transferring each successive batch to a clean saucepan.

Juice the lemon with the spinach. Stir the juice into the soup and season to taste. Heat through gently, if necessary.

Ladle the soup into bowls and top with a dollop of plain yogurt and sprinkling of chopped cilantro.

For creamy kale detox soup, heat 1 tablespoon coconut oil in a large saucepan. Add 1 peeled and chopped onion, 1 crushed garlic clove, a ¾ inch piece peeled and diced fresh ginger root, and ½ teaspoon turmeric and sauté for 4–5 minutes. Stir in 2 peeled and diced carrots and 2½ cups chopped kale. Pour in 1¾ cups coconut milk, the juice from 3 cups spinach, and 1 cup water, bring to a boil, and simmer for 12–15 minutes. Season to taste and serve sprinkled with chopped chives.

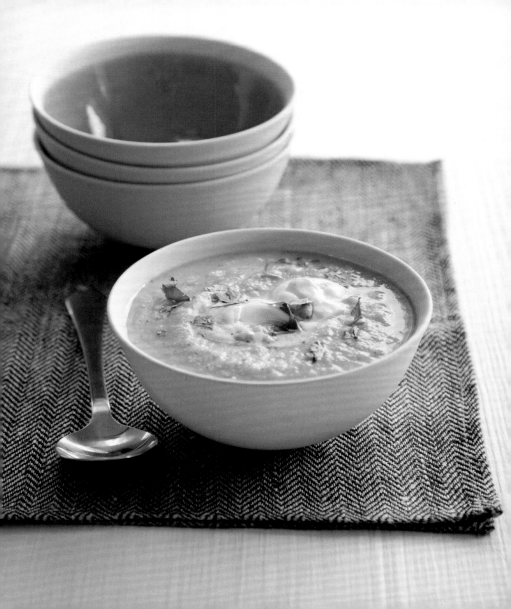

strawberry & melon soup

Serves **4**

2 **oranges**, coarsely peeled
1 **lemon**, coarsely peeled
1 small **cantaloupe**, peeled, seeded, and cut into chunks
2 cups hulled **strawberries**
1 teaspoon **honey** (optional)
2 tablespoons **plain yogurt**
2 tablespoon chopped **mint**

Juice the oranges with the lemon.

Transfer the juice to a food processor or blender, add the melon and strawberries, and process until smooth. Taste for sweetness and stir in the honey, if necessary. Chill for at least 1 hour, stirring in half the chopped mint 20 minutes before serving.

Ladle the soup into bowls, top with a dollop of plain yogurt, and sprinkle with the remaining chopped mint.

For warm berry soup, juice 6 apples. Pour the juice into a saucepan and add 2 cups assorted fresh berries, 1 cinnamon stick, and 2 cloves. Bring to a boil and simmer gently for 10 minutes. Process half the soup in a blender or food processor until smooth. Pour the processed soup back into the saucepan and stir into the remaining soup. Ladle the soup into bowls and serve with a dollop of plain yogurt.

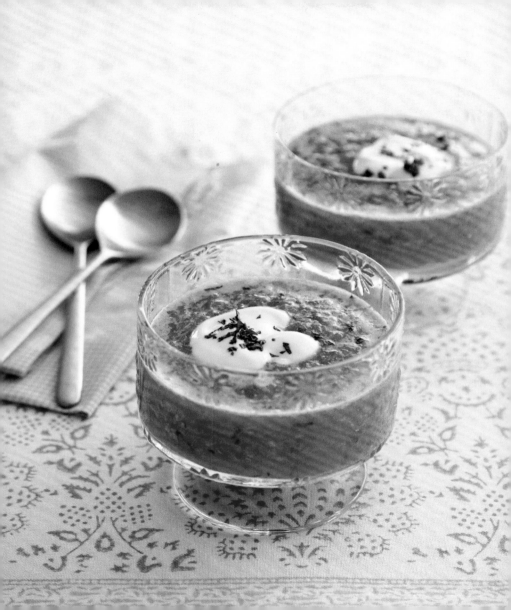

index

235

acknowledgments

Commissioning editor: Eleanor Maxfield
Editor: Pollyanna Poulter
Designers: Jaz Bahra and Tracy Killick
Production controller: Sarah Kramer

Octopus Publishing Group Octopus Publishing Group
Stephen Conroy 9 above, 16, 70, 128, 213, 217; Vanessa
Davies 101, 123; Janine Hosegood 105, 113, 61, 63, 65,
73, 79, 109, 121, 125, 131, 143, 157, 167, 173, 174, 200,
207; William Reavell 177; William Shaw 9 below, 10, 161,
171, 219, 223, 225, 227, 229; Ian Wallace 221. Shutterbroth
Evgeny Karandaev 11; Kesu 12; lola1960 13; Odua Images
15; Sabino Parente 14.